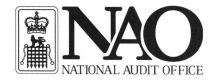

DEPARTMENT FOR ENVIRONMENT, FOOD AND RURAL AFFAIRS

Foot and Mouth Disease: Applying the Lessons

LONDON: The Stationery Office
£11.25

Ordered by the
House of Commons
to be printed on 31 January 2005

REPORT BY THE COMPTROLLER AND AUDITOR GENERAL | HC 184 Session 2004-2005 | 2 February 2005

This report has been prepared under Section 6 of the National Audit Act 1983 for presentation to the House of Commons in accordance with Section 9 of the Act.

John Bourn
**Comptroller and Auditor General
National Audit Office**

20 January 2005

The National Audit Office study team consisted of:

Tom Wallace, Sophie Buttle and Adam Crossley, under the direction of Joe Cavanagh

This report can be found on the National Audit Office web site at www.nao.org.uk

For further information about the National Audit Office please contact:

National Audit Office
Press Office
157-197 Buckingham Palace Road
Victoria
London
SW1W 9SP

Tel: 020 7798 7400

Email: enquiries@nao.gsi.gov.uk

CONTENTS

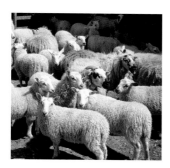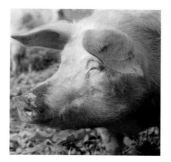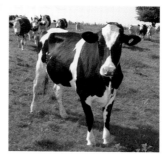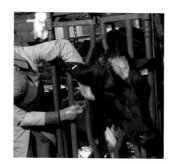

Photographs courtesy of Huw John and Alamy

EXECUTIVE SUMMARY

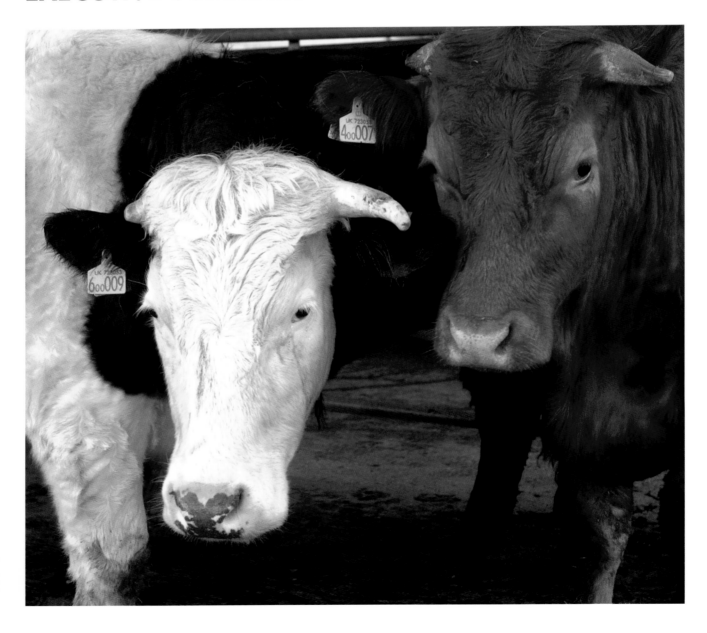

1   In March 2003 the House of Commons' Committee of Public Accounts (the Committee) reported on the 2001 outbreak of Foot and Mouth Disease.[1] The Committee made a number of recommendations to improve the management of future livestock epidemics by the Department for Environment, Food and Rural Affairs (the Department). This report examines the Government's response to the Committee in May 2003[2] and the progress made since then.

2   Throughout the report we have summarised our findings on the Department's preparations for a future outbreak using a traffic light analogy: a green light where the Committee's concerns have been addressed, amber where the Committee's concerns have been mostly addressed, and red where there is limited progress to report. **Figure 1** shows that overall we consider that the Department has implemented most of the actions promised to the Committee and has made good progress on the others since 2001.

3   Our main findings on the Department's preparations for a future outbreak are:

■   The Department has taken action, through improved animal health policies, to reduce the risk of an outbreak on the scale of 2001 - although further outbreaks can never be ruled out.

■   Preparedness for another outbreak is much improved – in terms of contingency planning, staff training, the availability of vaccination as an adjunct to culling, improved dialogue with stakeholders and standing arrangements with contractors to make resources available to fight any future outbreak. In addition,

1	Foot and Mouth Disease - traffic light analysis	
Report Ref	**Area**	**NAO evaluation**
Part 2	Preventing an outbreak of Foot and Mouth Disease	●
Part 3	Stopping an outbreak before it develops into a major epidemic	●
Part 4	Controlling the costs of a future outbreak	●

KEY

● Committee of Public Accounts' concerns addressed

● Concerns mostly addressed

● Progress is ongoing to address the Committee's concerns

Source: National Audit Office

the Department's disease control strategy is now better documented, and further research into disease control strategies is underway.

■   Some arrangements to control the cost of a future outbreak have been improved but new compensation arrangements await legislation, and discussions continue on establishing a levy scheme to share the cost of future outbreaks with the farming industry.

These findings are discussed in greater detail in the rest of this summary. We also examined how the Department has managed issues remaining from the 2001 outbreak: final payments to some contractors remain to be resolved.

---

1   *The 2001 Outbreak of Foot and Mouth Disease,* Committee of Public Accounts - Fifth Report 2002-03 HC 487 14 March 2003.
2   *Treasury Minutes on the Fifth, Sixth and Ninth Reports from the Committee of Public Accounts 2002-2003* Cm 5801 May 2003.

Background

4   Foot and Mouth Disease is one of the most highly infectious livestock diseases and it reduces significantly the productivity of infected animals. In 2001, the Department estimates that at least 57 separate farms were infected before the disease was first reported. The resulting epidemic was one of the largest and most costly animal disease outbreaks ever. At least six million animals were culled for disease control purposes or because of welfare problems resulting from the restrictions on animal movements.[3] The 2001 epidemic cost the taxpayer over £3 billion, including some £1.4 billion paid in compensation for culled animals. The total cost of the epidemic was offset by £350 million reimbursed by the European Commission.

5   Following the three inquiries into the outbreak by the Royal Society, Dr Iain Anderson (Lessons to be Learned enquiry) and the National Audit Office, the Department prepared a full response followed by a detailed action plan or "Route Map" in November 2002.[4] Following the report by the Committee of Public Accounts in March 2003, the Department also prepared a Treasury Minute[5] which sets out the Government's detailed response to the Committee's main findings and recommendations, and made a number of undertakings (Appendix 4). This report does not set out to repeat the information contained in these detailed documents, but rather to assess the progress made since the Committee's last report.

Main findings

The Department has acted to reduce the chance of another major livestock epidemic, but continued vigilance is essential

The Committee recommended improvements to biosecurity to reduce the chance of a future epidemic. The Treasury Minute set out details of the actions taken by the Department through its animal welfare strategy, including better controls over illegal meat imports and restrictions on the movement of animals.

6   **The Department has acted to reduce the chances of another outbreak.** The 2001 outbreak of Foot and Mouth Disease is most likely to have been caused by the illegal feeding of unprocessed swill containing meat contaminated with the Foot and Mouth Disease virus to pigs. The 2001 epidemic was made worse by the rapid dispersal of infected animals via livestock markets to farms in at least 16 counties, and to three other European countries, before the disease was reported. The Department's strategy for preventing new outbreaks includes the following main elements:

- **To reduce the chance of susceptible animals coming into contact with infectious material**, the feeding of waste food (swill) to pigs by farmers is now illegal and is likely to be detected quickly through farm inspections.

- **To encourage a greater use of disease prevention measures on farms**, the Department is encouraging farm assurance schemes and is working in partnership with different livestock sectors, vets, and agricultural colleges and others.

- **To slow the initial spread of the disease**, there are now greater routine restrictions on the movements of cattle and sheep and the gathering of animals at livestock markets. In addition, once an outbreak is confirmed, the Department will impose an immediate nationwide ban on all livestock movements.

- **To improve the identification and reporting of suspect cases**, the Department's animal health and welfare strategy will better co-ordinate farm inspections and encourage improved veterinary surveillance of farm animals.

- **To reduce the level of illegal meat and other agricultural imports, the Department has undertaken to spend a total of £25 million over three years, mostly to fund additional work at ports by Customs officers.** During 2003-04, Customs and local authorities seized 186 tonnes of illegal animal products, including an increase of over 100 per cent in seizures of illegal meat. Since the 2001 epidemic, the Department has attempted to maintain the high levels of public awareness of the risks from imported animal products. The National Audit Office is preparing a separate report on how HM Customs and Excise is seeking to stop illegal imports of agricultural products.

---

3   The figure excludes young animals which were valued with their mothers and not separately counted.
4   *Response to the Reports of the Foot and Mouth Disease Inquiries* Cm 5637 November 2002. The "Route Map" is available at http://www.defra.gov.uk/corporate/inquiries/response/index.htm
5   *Treasury Minutes on the Fifth, Sixth and Ninth Reports from the Committee of Public Accounts 2002-2003* Cm 5801 May 2003.

The Department is now better prepared to deal with a livestock epidemic

The Committee was concerned at weaknesses in contingency planning and recommended the Department improve its partnerships with rural stakeholders and the availability of key staff and veterinary resources; develop trigger points for involving the armed forces; and clarify its plans for vaccination. The Treasury Minute outlined the major changes made to the contingency plan since 2001 and the Department's efforts to reflect wider rural issues in its policy making.

7 **The Department has improved its capacity to deal with future outbreaks of livestock diseases and their contingency plan is one of the best available.** It now also includes explicit consideration of vaccination.[6] The Department has made considerable progress since February 2001 in improving its capacity and preparedness for combating another major disease outbreak including plans for increasing veterinary and other staff and other resources; over two hundred agreements with a wide range of suppliers of essential services; and capacity to deploy at least 50 vaccination teams within five days of confirmation of disease. The Department has carried out more than 30 exercises of varying scales to test their contingency plans including Exercise Hornbeam in June 2004 which involved more than 500 people. The introduction of an improved management information system – the Exotic Disease Control System – was delayed whilst the Department outsourced its information technology. In the meantime, the current Disease Control System, developed during the 2001 epidemic, is being maintained to ensure continued support for the Department's disease control activities in the interim.

8 **The new Foot and Mouth Disease contingency plan has been the subject of wide consultation with the farming industry, local authorities and other rural interest groups.** We compared this plan with a range of countries and we concluded that the UK plan is one of the best available, and the European Commission now considers that it complies with the latest European Directive. The Contingency Plan summarises the policies that would be immediately implemented, including the consideration of emergency vaccination. The plan is concerned primarily with the Department and central government decision-making processes and is not intended to cover local authorities, emergency services and other agencies such as tourist authorities who should have their own plans. The Department is currently working with local authorities to prepare a model local plan to ensure that that all those who would be involved in controlling the disease understand each other's roles and responsibilities and are able to operate in a co-ordinated and co-operative fashion.

9 **The Department's contingency plan does not include explicit consideration of a worst-case scenario.** However, the Department considers that the Plan provides for a wide range of scenarios. It has also commissioned work modelling a range of scenarios which will contribute to the Department's ability to increase veterinary and other resources to meet the needs of any realistic worst-case scenario.

10 **The Department will notify the Ministry of Defence on confirmation of disease, but the Ministry of Defence cannot guarantee the availability of troops in any civil emergency.** Thus the role of the military has not been specified in advance of an outbreak. The Committee recommended that the Department and the Ministry of Defence should plan for the early involvement of the military in future epidemics. However, the Treasury Minute argued that the specific aims and objectives of the troops are best agreed at the time of their deployment because the ability of the armed forces to participate in controlling a Foot and Mouth Disease epidemic is dependent on other commitments at the time of the outbreak. These arrangements are consistent with the national arrangements for civil contingencies, which have been the subject of a recent review by the Cabinet Office.[7] The Department considers that this arrangement together with Military Liaison Officers being in the National and Local Disease Control Centres from the outset retains a degree of flexibility to use the military to assist in dealing with unforeseen circumstances in a future outbreak. It also believes that relevant leadership and communications skills which the military brought to the 2001 operation are being maintained within the Department by inclusion in the contingency plan and through regular realistic exercises. Other areas where military expertise played a major part such as carcase disposal logistics will be managed through contracts with commercial firms.

---

6   We compared the UK contingency plan and plans published by six other countries and with guidance from the European Commission and others (Appendix 6 and paragraph 3.4).

7   *Dealing with Disaster* (revised 3rd edition) Cabinet Office Civil Contingencies Secretariat ISBN 1-874447-42-X.

11   As promised in the Treasury Minute, the latest contingency plan includes details of the Department's proposals for vaccination – but the decision to use will be a complex one. The latest European Directive on Foot and Mouth Disease requires that all animals on infected farms or otherwise exposed to the disease should be culled. Emergency vaccination of animals is allowed as an additional measure. The Department can now begin vaccination within five days - as soon as stocks of vaccine can be made up from frozen antigen. However, the decision whether or not to vaccinate commercial livestock in any particular area is a very complex one and would have to be taken in the face of many uncertainties. The Foot and Mouth Disease contingency plan includes a "decision tree" setting out internationally recognised criteria for decisions on vaccination including, for example, the density of livestock in the affected area. Neither the European Directive, nor most of the other countries' contingency plans we examined, contain specific circumstances which would trigger vaccination, and most plans include less detail on how the optimum control strategy is to be decided on. In June 2004 the Department also published a paper on the role of vaccination in any future outbreak, and held a major exercise in June 2004 which resulted in a decision to use vaccination to control the hypothetical outbreak.

12   Vaccination is likely to feature more prominently in the response to a future outbreak, and the supply of vaccine has been substantially increased. Plans to vaccinate up to 180,000 cattle in 2001 were not used largely due to the opposition expected from farmers and the food industry. The Department has, since 2001, engaged with a wide range of stakeholders on issues arising from the use of emergency vaccination against Foot and Mouth Disease. These discussions have involved the full food chain – from producers through to retailers and ensured that stakeholder's views were taken account of during negotiations on the new European Union Directive on Foot and Mouth Disease in 2003. Further work is currently underway to address particular concerns of the dairy and meat industry on the impact of Foot and Mouth Disease control measures especially emergency vaccination.

13   On supply, the Department has substantially increased the UK stocks of antigen used to prepare vaccine since 2001. Foot and Mouth Disease is a highly variable virus. The UK vaccine bank now holds sufficient antigens to make in total over 20 million doses of Foot and Mouth Disease vaccine. The minimum quantity of any one of the nine strains of the virus most likely to be involved in a future outbreak is around 500,000 doses. Although widespread vaccination of sheep and pigs is unlikely to be beneficial, there are over 10 million cattle in the United Kingdom. The Department formally reviews vaccine stocks annually on the basis of independent advice from the Institute of Animal Health and additional purchases will be made if that is justified by the international situation. In the event of another UK outbreak, some further vaccine supplies may be available from international stocks such as the European Community's Vaccine Bank and from manufacturers, but the latter cannot be guaranteed.

14   The European Union policy on the control of Foot and Mouth Disease is to cull all susceptible animals in an infected place and any dangerous contacts. Whether or not vaccination is employed in a future epidemic, the immediate cull of all susceptible animals on infected premises along with the rapid identification and slaughter of any animals that have been exposed to infection (dangerous contacts), through human contacts, vehicle and animal movements or airborne spread, remains the primary method of control both in the United Kingdom and throughout the European Union. There will not be an automatic cull of animals on neighbouring (contiguous) premises - unless a potential route of infection is identified by veterinarians. However, if initial efforts to control the epidemic are unsuccessful, and vaccination is not feasible, a more extensive cull of animals on neighbouring farms, as in 2001, remains a possibility because animals on contiguous premises are at greater risk of infection by virtue of their proximity to infected animals.

15   The Department made available all its data on the 2001 outbreak to independent academic researchers during 2003. Scientific opinion on the relative effectiveness of vaccination and cull of contiguous premises is divided, and the subject remains controversial with different scientific teams producing widely different conclusions. In January 2004 the Department commissioned a major cost benefit analysis of different disease control strategies, including vaccination and contiguous cull, using improved computer models. Initial findings will be reported early in 2005.

The Department has improved controls over the costs of future epidemics

The Committee was concerned that better benchmarks were needed for assessing compensation paid for culled animals, prices for key services should be agreed in advance with suppliers, and better control should be exercised over the costs of cleansing infected premises. The Treasury Minute outlined the progress made on these areas by May 2003 and promised a range of public consultations on detailed proposals by 2004.

16 **The Department has issued extended guidance to valuers which is significantly better than that used in 2001 but has not provided benchmark valuations**. The Department has drawn up a list of 280 approved valuers who will be paid by the hour rather than by a percentage of the valuation as in 2001. Other improvements made since 2001 include the appointment of independent monitors to assess the valuations undertaken by approved valuers and to advise the Department on any additional instructions that need to be issued to the approved valuers in an outbreak. The extended guidance includes a range of factors which the approved valuers are expected to include (for example the valuation of hefted sheep - specialised flocks occupying hill or other pasturage), and the need for improved documentation to support the valuations. However, the guidance does not provide detailed instructions on how valuers should reach their assessments because the Department expects professionally qualified valuers to be competent and believes that further detail would undermine the independence of the valuation process. The Department also believes that benchmarks are not readily available for dairy cattle and pedigree animals. In addition, valuers who give significant cause for concern will be removed from the approved list.

17 **In October 2003, the Department consulted on a new compensation scheme for all notifiable animal diseases which would apply standard rates based on average market values prior to the outbreak**. In addition, owners of higher value animals would have the option of having them independently valued, at their own expense, prior to the outbreak, and the valuation agreed by the Department. This scheme would reduce the scope for disputes over compensation delaying the cull of infected animals and help to ensure that above average animals are valued realistically.

18 **The Department has improved its guidance on the costs of cleansing and disinfection**. In 2001, cleansing and disinfection of farms cost the taxpayer an average of £30,000 per farm. In the Netherlands farmers were required to carry out much of this work at their own expense. Neither country experienced re-emergence of the disease. The European Commission was critical of the controls exercised over the costs of cleansing and disinfection in 2001 and recently disallowed 80 per cent of the Department's claim for £209 million. The latest Departmental guidance requires cleansing and disinfection to be proportionate to the risk, and requires staff to use their judgement to assess what should be cleansed and disinfected on an individual farm. The Department does not consider that benchmark or maximum values would be effective – and could lead to excessive work being done on low risk sites.

19 **Proposals for a scheme to share the costs of a future animal disease outbreak between the farming industry and the taxpayer are expected soon**. The Department's proposals for an industry levy scheme and other charges to farmers have been delayed pending decisions on the regulation of farming and the cumulative impact of policy changes, including reform of the Common Agricultural Policy. The Department is finalising a proposed scheme for public consultation which is expected to cover all major animal diseases and ensure that the industry contributes towards the Department's animal health expenditure and the costs of dealing with major disease outbreaks. The cost of controlling a future outbreak will continue to be borne by the taxpayer until the proposed compulsory industry levy scheme is in place. The new scheme may include an element related to compliance with good practice in biosecurity.

The final cost of the 2001 epidemic for UK taxpayers is yet to be determined

20   The final contribution by the European Union towards the Department's £3 billion cost of the 2001 outbreak – some £350 million - was significantly less than the £960 million claimed. The European Commission generally reimburses 60 per cent of Member State's eligible expenditure including compensation for compulsory slaughter of animals and certain "other costs" of disease eradication process (for example, the cleansing of infected premises). Following the outbreak, in line with European legislation, the Department submitted three claims for re-imbursement (two claims for compensation costs and one for 'other costs'). These three claims amounted to some £960 million. Following a review of a sample of high value compensation claims, together with other indicators of the value of culled animals, the Commission concluded that farmers were compensated on average between two and three times the market value. The Department accepts that the compensation system in use during the emergency was flawed but believes that the Commission's conclusions overstate the extent of the problem. In addition, the European Commission conducted a detailed review of the UK's "other costs" claim. The Commission initially offered to pay £230 million in settlement of all three claims. However, following discussions with the Department and a re-examination of their work, the Commission revised the amount refundable to £350 million (£253 million for animals culled and £97 million for 'other costs').

The Committee was concerned that the Department should seek recovery where it believes it was overcharged [by contractors] in 2001. The Treasury Minute outlined the Department's approach to settling disputed invoices through negotiation, mediation, litigation and formal overpayment procedures.

21   The Department has paid 97 per cent of the invoices submitted by contractors since 2001 but has not yet finalised payments to 57 contractors. The Department has spent over £25 million on professional services to investigate invoices for the £1.3 billion expenditure on goods, services and works arising out of the 2001 outbreak; but it estimates that this has produced savings for the taxpayer of at least £57 million.

- The Department has completed an initial review of invoices submitted by 108 of the 130 largest suppliers. Final payments have been agreed in 73 cases, valued at £444 million, by negotiation or through formal dispute resolution procedures which have saved £40 million. In the other 35 cases alternative dispute resolution procedures, and possibly litigation, are likely to be needed to resolve the difficult issues involved. The first cases to be tested in court were heard during 2003. The first judgement in January 2004 was a mixed result for the Department. Nine cases are now in the High Court and one case is the subject of ongoing Police investigation. A further case has been referred to the Special Compliance Office of the Inland Revenue as the relevant investigating authority.

- The Department expects to complete its initial review of invoices submitted by the remaining 22 suppliers by the end of March 2005 or earlier. In the cases where a final settlement has not been reached, the Department has already agreed reductions of a further £17 million.

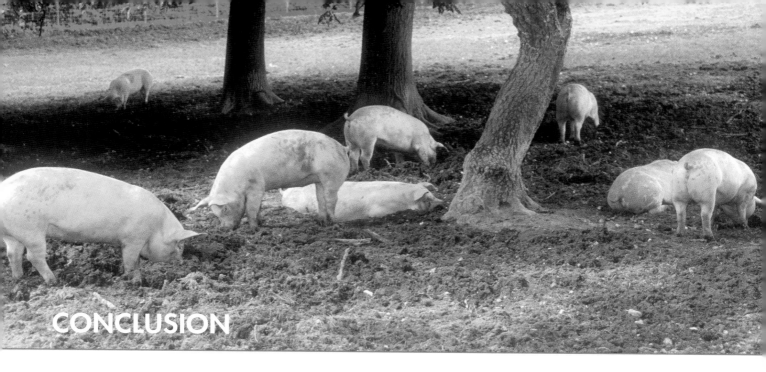

CONCLUSION

22   Although good progress has been made since 2001 on most of the recommendations made by the Committee following the 2001 epidemic, the Department recognises that further work is needed in some key areas:

■   The Department's contingency plan is focused on central government, but it is now working with other public bodies such as local authorities to agree roles and responsibilities to be recorded in complementary plans.

■   The Department has commissioned a cost benefit analysis of alternative disease control policies and made its data on 2001 available to independent researchers – results are awaited and will thereafter be reflected in disease control strategies and contingency plans.

■   The Department is reviewing its Information Technology support in any future outbreak to determine a revised programme for the introduction of essential improvements.

■   The cost of controlling livestock disease outbreaks currently falls predominantly on the taxpayer rather than the industry. The Department has proposed an animal health levy scheme to share the burden in future, and it will report the findings from its consultation to Parliament.

■   The Department is developing a new compensation system which will remove the need to use independent valuers to value animals prior to their cull. However, this system will require primary legislation and is unlikely to be in place until 2008.

■   The Department is continuing to seek negotiated settlements with contractors which it believes have overcharged for services provided during 2001 and will consider legal action where necessary. Some 3 per cent of invoices remain to be settled.

PART ONE
Introduction

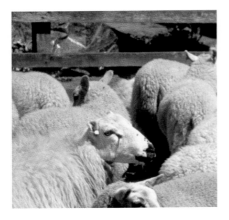
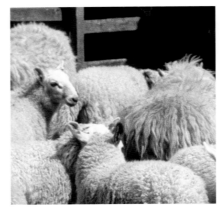
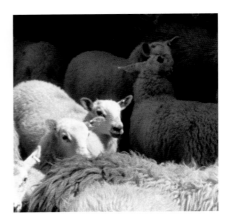
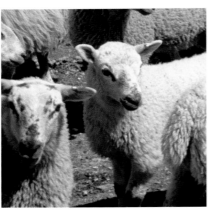
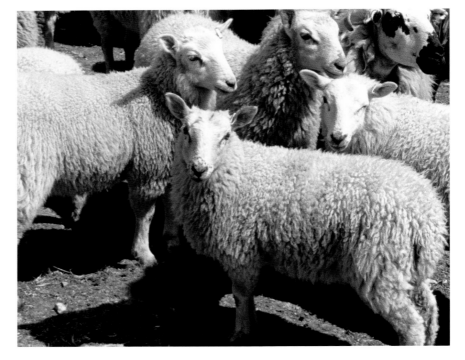

1.1 This Part of the Report sets out the health and financial risks from Foot and Mouth Disease; the role of the Department for Environment, Food and Rural Affairs (the Department); and the scope and aims of our examination.

Foot and Mouth Disease is highly infectious and economically damaging

1.2 Foot and Mouth Disease (Appendix 2) is one of the most infectious animal diseases, capable of developing rapidly into a major epidemic affecting thousands of farms. The scale of the 2001 epidemic was unprecedented in the United Kingdom and it led to the culling of over 4 million animals, along with their young, for disease control purposes. A further 2 million animals were culled on welfare grounds due to restrictions on animal movements during the epidemic. The cost to the Department was over £2.7 billion (**Figure 2**). The wider costs to rural stakeholders is less certain, but may have been some £5 billion, mainly due to the adverse effect of the outbreak on international and domestic tourism (between £2.7 and £3.2 billion). However, the epidemic also caused some £355 million in uncompensated losses by agricultural producers - about 20 per cent of the estimated net income from farming in 2001.

2	Estimated cost of the 2001 epidemic to the Department for Environment, Food and Rural Affairs

The final cost of the 2001 epidemic of Foot and Mouth Disease is around £2.7 billion. Some £52 million of invoices are the subject of dispute (see Part 5).

Type of cost	Estimated final expenditure (£ million)
Compensation payments for animals culled	1,369
Payments to contractors	1,279
Other costs	412
Total	3,060
Less contribution from the European Union	(350)
Net cost to the Department	**2,710**

Sources: National Audit Office, Department for Environment, Food and Rural Affairs

The Department has primary responsibility for animal health

1.3 The main responsibilities of the Department's Animal Health and Welfare Directorate are:

- To protect the public's interest in relation to environmental impacts and health and ensure high standards of animal health and welfare.

- In consultation with the devolved administrations, to represent UK interests at the international level, in particular within the European Union.

1.4 The Department's State Veterinary Service has a range of responsibilities including dealing with outbreaks of notifiable diseases, carrying out welfare visits to farms and markets, and advising farmers on disease prevention and requirements for importing and exporting. Other major agencies with responsibilities are local authorities, the Food Standards Agency and the Meat Hygiene Service, Her Majesty's Customs and Excise[8], and Port Health Authorities **(Figure 3)**.

We looked at the Department's response to previous recommendations of the Committee of Public Accounts

1.5 Following the three official inquiries carried out by the Royal Society, Dr Iain Anderson (Lessons to be Learned Inquiry) and the National Audit Office, the Department responded[9] and prepared an action plan, or "route map"[10], in November 2002. Following the report by the Committee of Public Accounts in March 2003, (the Committee or PAC) a Treasury Minute[11] set out the Government's detailed response to the Committee's main findings and recommendations and includes a range of actions promised for 2003 and 2004 (Appendix 4). This report does not repeat the information contained in these detailed documents, but seeks to assess the progress made since the Committee's last report.

1.6 We examined the progress made by the Department to:

- minimise the chances of a future outbreak of Foot and Mouth Disease (Part 2 of this report)

- prevent any future outbreak becoming an epidemic (Part 3); and

- control the costs of future outbreaks (Part 4).

We also examined the Department's progress in finalising the cost of the 2001 outbreak (Part 5).

1.7 We used a range of methods (see Appendix 1). We consulted widely with groups affected by the 2001 epidemic. We received 35 submissions from various stakeholders (see Appendix 5). We also interviewed key parties involved in operational aspects of animal disease control and outbreaks. We researched contingency plans drawn up by other State Veterinary Services and compared the UK contingency plan with guidance from the United Nation's Food and Agricultural Organisation and European Commission Directives. We also discussed our findings with an expert panel and with the Royal Society, which published a review of progress made on recommendations arising from its 2002 report *Infectious Diseases in Livestock,* in December 2004, and our report reflects these discussions.

---

8   From 1 April 2005 Her Majesty's Revenue and Customs.
9   *Response to the Reports of the Foot and Mouth Disease Inquiries* Cm 5637 November 2002.
10   The "Route Map" is available at http://www.defra.gov.uk/corporate/inquiries/response/index.htm
11   *Treasury Minutes on the Fifth, Sixth and Ninth Reports from the Committee of Public Accounts 2002-2003* Cm 5801 May 2003.

3 Organisations with responsibility for Foot and Mouth Disease in England

A wide range of public bodies have a role in preventing, or responding to, an outbreak of Foot and Mouth Disease.

Reducing illegal imports of meat	Improving Animal Health	Dealing with a disease outbreak
Department for Environment, Food and Rural Affairs (Lead Department)		
Policy advice to Ministers on imports of animal products, animal health and disease		
Represents UK interests at EU and internationally		
Sets legal framework		

Reducing illegal imports of meat	Improving Animal Health	Dealing with a disease outbreak
State Veterinary Service		
Assistance to Customs and Port Health officials	Farm Inspections	Contingency planning
	Disease surveillance	Cull & disposal of animals on all affected premises
		Cleansing and disinfection of farms

HM Customs & Excise		Environment Agency
Anti-smuggling controls on illegal imports		Monitoring of disposal
Support of Port Health Authorities		Environmental assessment and advice
International post		

	170 Local authorities	
	Livestock identification and records	
Public health inspections at restaurants, butchers etc	Inspections at markets, farms and abattoirs	Supporting disease control on infected farms
	Carry out checks on livestock vehicles (with police)	Restrictions on infected areas

Food Standards Agency (inc Meat Hygiene Service)		Cabinet Office
		Civil Contingencies Secretariat
Guidance to local and port health authorities	National inspection and enforcement service at 1,400 licensed slaughterhouses, cutting plants and cold stores	Inter-departmental cooperation
Coordination of intelligence		**Armed Forces**
		Support to the civil authorities

62 Port Health Authorities	39 Police forces	
Import checks on livestock and animal products	Livestock vehicles checks (with local authorities)	Public order duties
		Enforcing warrants

Source: National Audit Office

PART TWO

The Department has acted to reduce the chance of another major livestock epidemic

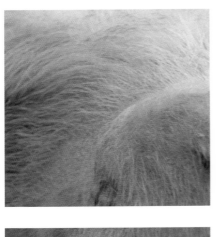
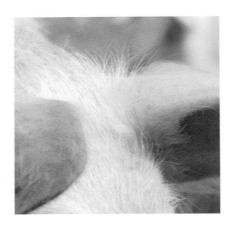
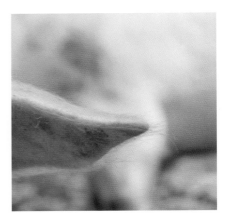
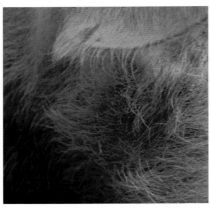
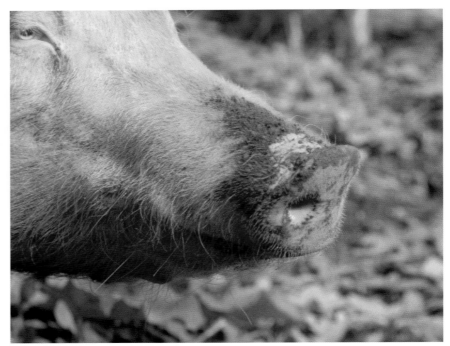

2.1 In this Part of the report, we examine how the Department has assessed the risks of another outbreak of Foot and Mouth Disease and the measures introduced to reduce the risk of a major epidemic. **Figure 4** summarises our findings on these issues using a traffic light analogy.

The Animal Health and Welfare Strategy provides a co-ordinated programme to reduce the risk of outbreaks

2.2 The Department's preparation for a future outbreak of Foot and Mouth Disease is part of its Animal Health and Welfare Strategy the aim of which is "to safeguard and improve the health and welfare of kept animals and protect society, the economy, and the environment from the effect of animal diseases". The Strategy incorporates a range of initiatives **(Figure 5 overleaf)** which the Department believes will significantly reduce the risk of future livestock epidemics. Some of these initiatives are described in the sections which follow.

4	Traffic light analysis - Preventing an outbreak of Foot and Mouth Disease	
Report Ref	**Area**	**NAO evaluation**
2.4-2.5	Preventing the import of infected meat products	◐
2.3	Removing infected matter from animal feedstuffs	●
2.6-2.7	Early recognition of an initial Foot and Mouth Disease case	◐
2.8	Preventing the movement of infected animals	●
2.9-2.10	Tracing the movement of potentially infected animals	●

KEY

● Committee of Public Account's concerns addressed

◐ Concerns mostly addressed

● Progress is ongoing to address the Committee's concerns

Source: National Audit Office

5 The Animal Health and Welfare Strategy includes a range of major initiatives which should reduce the risk of future livestock epidemics

The Department's preparation for a future outbreak of Foot and Mouth Disease is part of an overall Animal Health and Welfare Strategy.

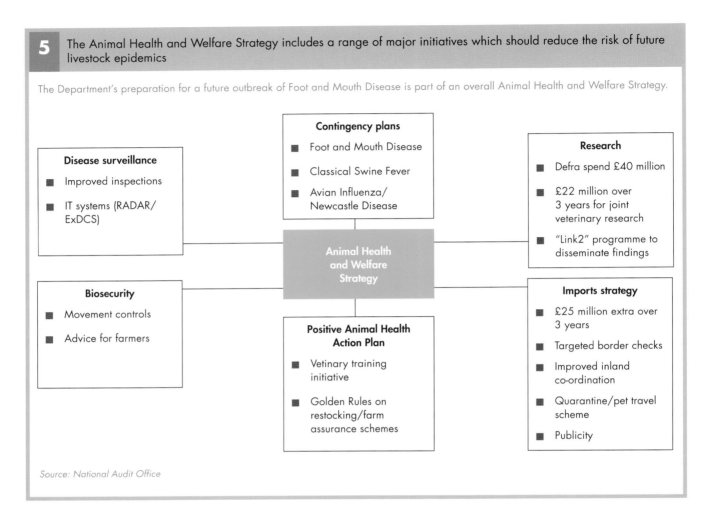

Disease surveillance
- Improved inspections
- IT systems (RADAR/ExDCS)

Biosecurity
- Movement controls
- Advice for farmers

Contingency plans
- Foot and Mouth Disease
- Classical Swine Fever
- Avian Influenza/Newcastle Disease

Animal Health and Welfare Strategy

Positive Animal Health Action Plan
- Vetinary training initiative
- Golden Rules on restocking/farm assurance schemes

Research
- Defra spend £40 million
- £22 million over 3 years for joint veterinary research
- "Link2" programme to disseminate findings

Imports strategy
- £25 million extra over 3 years
- Targeted border checks
- Improved inland co-ordination
- Quarantine/pet travel scheme
- Publicity

Source: National Audit Office

UK defences against illegal meat imports have been strengthened but can never guarantee that disease will not enter the country

Public Accounts Committee (PAC) main finding: "The Department should ensure that the [import] measures adopted in the United Kingdom are at least the equal of those elsewhere in the developed world, including Australia, New Zealand and the United States."

2.3 The 1967 Foot and Mouth Disease outbreak was caused by infected lamb imported legally from Argentina, which was then fed to pigs. Whilst it is not possible to be certain of the source of the 2001 epidemic, it is most likely to have been the inclusion of illegally imported meat in pigswill, and the failure of a farmer to heat-treat the swill to inactivate the virus. The feeding of swill to pigs was rare in 2001 and since May 2001 has been banned.[12] Farms are subject to a range of inspections both by the Department and local authorities and it is unlikely that the equipment needed to distribute swill to animals could remain undetected for any length of time. Thus the chance that commercial livestock will come into contact with active virus from either legal or illegal meat has been substantially reduced.

2.4 The Veterinary Laboratories Agency estimates that between 65kg and 565kg of meat contaminated with live Foot and Mouth Disease virus is smuggled into Great Britain annually (0.001 per cent of all illegally imported meat) either for personal consumption or for resale commercially. The wide margin in the estimate reflects the lack of data currently available. In 2003-04, 186 tonnes of illegal animal products were seized by Customs and local authorities – 70 per cent more than in the previous year. Within this figure, seizures of illegal meat increased by over 100 per cent from 31 tonnes in 2002-03 to 73 tonnes in 2003-04.

12   Animal By-Products (Amendment) Order 2001.

2.5 Following a major study conducted by the Machinery of Government Secretariat in the Cabinet Office[13], anti-smuggling controls for meat and other agricultural products at ports and airports has been the responsibility of a single agency – HM Customs and Excise - since April 2003. The Department has allocated £25 million across the three financial years 2003-04 to 2005-06 to raise awareness of, and enforce restrictions, relating to illegal meat and animal imports. This funding is distributed between the Department, the Food Standards Agency and HM Customs and Excise, with the bulk going to the last of these. The National Audit Office is preparing a separate report on how HM Customs and Excise is seeking to reduce illegal imports of agricultural produce.

Awareness of animal disease is high in the farming community but the Department needs to ensure that industry does not become complacent

PAC conclusion (iii): "the Department should aim for a high degree of awareness of animal disease in the farming industry ... [and] educate farmers and vets about diseases they might not have encountered."

2.6 In the 2001 epidemic, at least 57 farms became infected before the disease was reported to the Department. The Department's modelling has confirmed its view that a key variable in determining the overall size of a Foot and Mouth Disease epidemic is the initial delay in reporting disease signs to the veterinary authorities. In a disease as infectious as Foot and Mouth Disease, the Department's normal surveillance activities and the on-farm inspections by the State Veterinary Service or local authorities are unlikely to detect an initial case prior to its spread to other premises. The onus is on the farmer and veterinarian in regular contact with livestock to report suspicious cases. By the end of the 2001 epidemic, 72 per cent of Foot and Mouth Disease cases were detected in this way – although three quarters of all reports proved to be false alarms.

2.7 There is a legal requirement on livestock farmers and private veterinarians to report a range of livestock diseases to the State Veterinary Service. In 2003 22 cases of suspected Foot and Mouth Disease were reported compared to an average of 6 a year before the 2001 outbreak. The British Veterinary Association considers that although Foot and Mouth Disease in cattle and pigs would be obvious to most farmers, in sheep it is a challenge even for experienced veterinary surgeons to spot the disease due to its mild signs and its similarity with more common ailments. The Department provides non-technical information and pictures of signs of Foot and Mouth Disease on its website[14] and the State Veterinary Service Journal has published detailed technical advice on the diagnosis of Foot and Mouth Disease in sheep, aimed at a professional audience. In addition, the Department's Animal Health and Welfare Strategy includes a Positive Health Action Plan, published in September 2004, which sets out how the Department is working with interested parties to promote wider adoption of farm health planning and disease recognition.

The Department is improving the tracking of animals

PAC main finding: "the Department should have imposed a national movement ban from the first day..."

2.8 In future, the Department intends to impose an immediate ban on all livestock movements throughout the UK immediately an outbreak is confirmed. In addition, in August 2003 the Department announced that the six-day whole farm standstill following sheep and cattle movements, imposed after the 2001 epidemic, would be permanent except for some limited exemptions. This will help to prevent normal commercial movements creating many mini-epidemics before the disease is first reported. The organisations that we consulted generally supported the permanent restrictions, but some expressed concern that the national movement ban should be lifted as early as possible once the extent of infected areas is known.

---

13 *The Organisation Of The Government's Controls Of Imports Of Animals, Fish, Plants and their Products.* Machinery of Government Secretariat, The Cabinet Office, November 2002.

14 See www.defra.gov.uk/footandmouth/about/clinical.htm

PAC conclusion (viii): "[the Department] should institute effective checks for unmarked animals and penalise those who deal in them."

2.9 Primary responsibility for checking animal identification and movements rests with trading standards staff in 170 local authorities in England and Wales; the Rural Payments Agency also inspects cattle holdings.[15] During 2003 the Department introduced a trial Framework Agreement with 85 local authorities, and by August 2004 160 authorities were covered. The Framework provides more reliable and regular reporting on the results of local authority enforcement. Early results show that in 2003 these 85 authorities had undertaken 73,444 inspections. In all, some 182 prosecutions were initiated in 2003 for animal movement and livestock identification infringements. Where legal action has been completed, 38 prosecutions for offences involving cattle were successful, 34 initiated by local authorities and 4 by the Department, and 2 cases have been withdrawn and 2 others are pending appeal.

2.10 In March 2004 the Department participated in a traffic exercise involving 43 police forces to check commercial vehicles. Some 23 per cent of the vehicles transporting animals were found to have breached livestock movement restrictions or other animal welfare requirements, including failure to cleanse and disinfect vehicles and incorrect movement documents. Further similar exercises are planned with all offenders considered for prosecution, caution or warnings as appropriate.

---

15   In February 2004, the Committee of Public Accounts took evidence on the effectiveness of the Department's livestock tracking systems. (House of Commons Committee of Public Accounts Identifying and tracking livestock in England. Twenty–seventh Report of Session 2003–04.) This report does not return to all the issues covered by the Committee but focuses on checks and penalties against those who seek to circumvent the rules on animal identification and tracking.

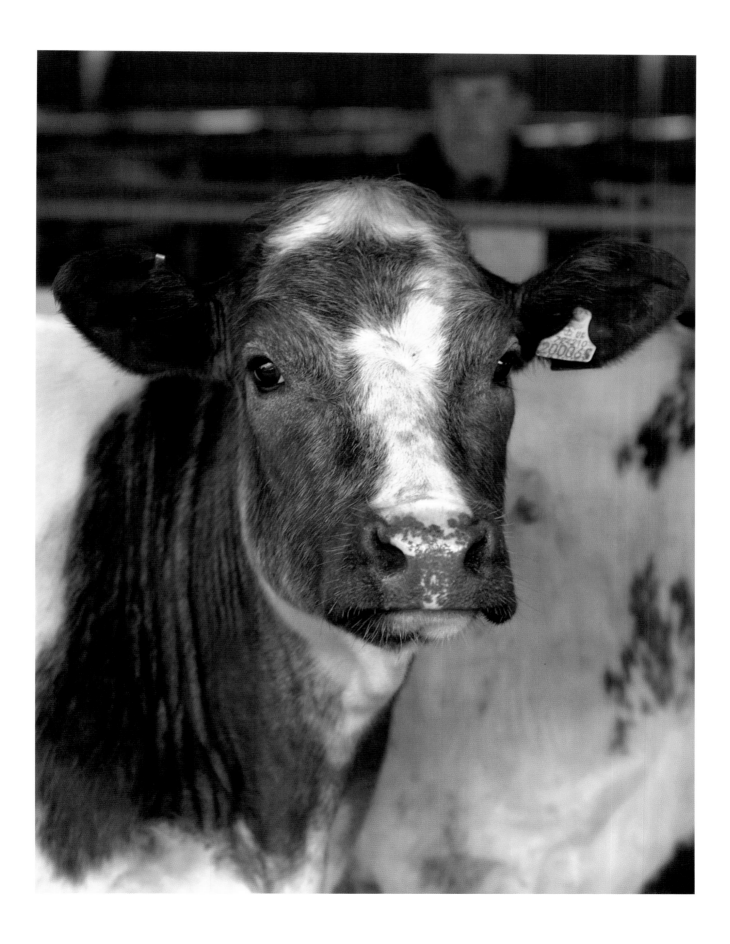

PART THREE

The Department is now better prepared to prevent an outbreak becoming an epidemic

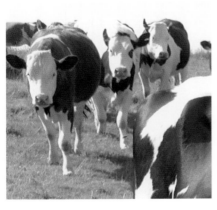
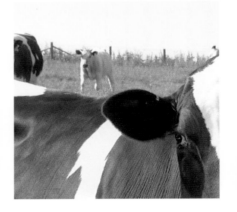
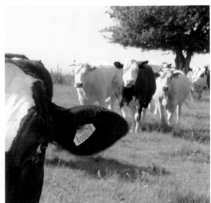
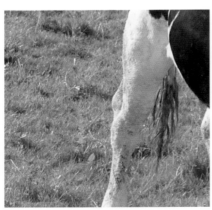
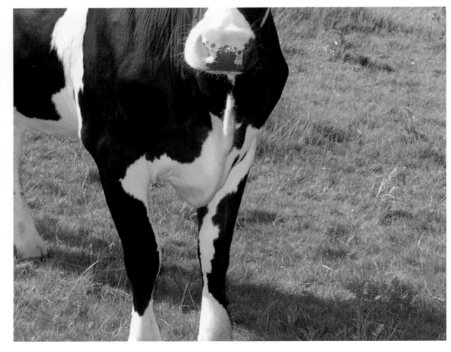

3.1 In the event of a livestock disease outbreak, the Department is the lead agency with responsibility for co-ordinating the efforts of national and local agencies in England and, in consultation with the Welsh Assembly Government, in Wales. The State Veterinary Service provides a service throughout Great Britain, with each national administration retaining responsibility for policy and operational matters.

3.2 This part of the report examines the adequacy of the Department's preparations for a future epidemic in the light of recommendations made by the Committee of Public Accounts, the revised European Union Directive on Foot and Mouth Disease, and guidance issued by the United Nations Food and Agricultural Organisation and other international agencies. This part also examines the availability of key staff resources and the preparations for the use of vaccination in a future epidemic. **Figure 6** summarises our findings on these issues using a traffic light analogy.

Since 2001 the Foot and Mouth Disease contingency plan has been updated and improved and compares well internationally

3.3 Prior to the 2001 epidemic, the Department had developed a contingency plan to deal with an outbreak of Foot and Mouth Disease. The plan fully complied with the existing European Union directive on Foot and Mouth Disease. A more detailed contingency plan was published following the 2001 epidemic, incorporating much of the lessons learnt during the emergency and changes in the European Directive. The current contingency plan (version 4), was published in March 2004. The plan summarises the policies that would be implemented immediately including consideration of emergency vaccination, and it includes a Veterinary Risk Assessment for Rights of Way Closure, a Decision Tree for Control Strategies and a Disease Control (Slaughter) Protocol. The plan has been subject to annual review as required by the *Animal Health Act 2002* and includes information as shown in **Figure 7**.

6   Traffic light analysis - preventing an outbreak becoming a major epidemic

Report Ref	Area	NAO evaluation
3.3-3.4, 3.9, 3.21	Realistic contingency plans are available for all major diseases	●
3.5-3.7	Rural stakeholders understand their role	◐
3.22-3.26	Sufficient veterinary resources available for disease control	●
3.27	Clarity over when to call in armed forces	●
3.10-3.16	Clear plans for vaccination agreed	●
3.17-19	Decision on a contiguous cull based on experience from 2001	◐
3.20	Sufficient resources are available for disposal of culled animals	●
3.26, 3.29	Defra is prepared for emergency response	●
3.28	IT support systems are available	●

KEY

● Committee of Public Account's concerns addressed

◐ Concerns mostly addressed

● Progress is ongoing to address the Committee's concerns

Source: National Audit Office

7   The Department has a detailed contingency plan for dealing with an outbreak of Foot and Mouth Disease

The Department has developed a detailed contingency plan setting out the likely response to a future outbreak of Foot and Mouth Disease. The full plan is available at www.defra.gov.uk.

The plan sets out details of:

■ Organisational structures at national, regional and local levels

■ Disease control policies including vaccination

■ Provision of staff

■ Liaison arrangements with the Environment Agency, local authorities, Government Offices in the Regions, police and farming organisations

■ Biosecurity guidance

■ Protection Zones and Surveillance Zones

■ Permanent Expert Group to advise government

■ Communications plan

■ Mobile team to quality assure local processes

Source: Department for Environment Food and Rural Affairs

3.4 We compared the Department's contingency plan against those prepared by a range of countries, best practice derived from the European Union Directive, a model contingency plan produced by the Food and Agricultural Organisation of the United Nations and guidance prepared by AVIS, a consortium of groups involved in animal health issues (see Appendix 6). We concluded that the UK contingency plan was one of the best available, giving a good level of detail on a range of the key issues and unlike the others we examined now includes explicit consideration of vaccination. In 2003 the UK contingency plan was reviewed by the European Commission who found that it complied with the latest European Directive.

The new contingency plan has been the subject of widespread consultation with rural stakeholders and continues to be developed

PAC conclusion (i): "the Department should bring all interested parties on board and discuss its contingency plans with central and local government, farmers and other major stakeholders. "

3.5 Each of the annual revisions of the contingency plan since 2001 has been the subject of extensive consultation. Non-farming stakeholders, emergency services and local authorities whom we contacted during the study expressed satisfaction with the Department's consultation process. The tourist industry welcomed the clarification on closure of footpaths – which will normally now be restricted to 3 kilometres around premises where disease is confirmed. *VisitBritain* suggested that the contingency plan should set out in more detail the arrangements for informing potential visitors to the country about the nature of the restrictions and the responsibilities of visitors. The Department has included a much extended communication strategy in the latest revision of the contingency plan.

3.6 Some concern has been expressed by our consultees about the lack of clearly defined roles for supporting agencies within the Contingency Plan. However, the plan is intended for central government and does not extend to other agencies. Nevertheless, the Department is working with other public bodies including representatives of Local Authorities Co-ordinators of Regulatory Services (LACoRS), the Local Government Association, the Environment Agency, the Association of Chief Police Officers, and the Health Protection Agency to agree their roles and responsibilities in a future epidemic. Already this work is leading to an improved understanding between the Department and other agencies and hence a more consistent response across the country.

PAC main finding: "contingency plans should not only address farming but also the difficulties likely to be experienced by other industries. The focus on farming interests, important as these are, needs to be complemented by greater recognition of wider rural and national concerns. "

3.7 As with the other contingency plans we examined, the UK plan covers mainly the immediate disease control arrangements. For a substantial outbreak, the plan requires the Department to activate the Cabinet Office Civil Contingencies Committee which will be responsible for the assessment of the wider impact of the developing outbreak and developing cross-departmental strategies, in particular, for issues affecting the wider UK economy. More generally, the Department was created in 2001 to ensure that policies for farming are developed in the context of wider rural and national concerns. This is reflected in the inclusion in the contingency plan of the protocols on rights of way closures and the establishment of the Rural Stress Action Plan Working Group. In addition, the Rural Affairs Forum for England was set up in January 2002 to bring together representatives of a wide range of organisations interested in rural issues.

The Department carries out regular tests of its contingency plans, including a major exercise in June 2004

PAC main finding: "stakeholders in affected industries should be fully consulted about contingency plans; and should participate in the simulation exercises carried out to test them. The Department also needs to build stronger and more confident partnerships with other relevant bodies … so as to make better use of their expertise and resources."

3.8 European legislation requires member states to carry out two major exercises every five years. Since the end of the 2001 epidemic, the Department has carried out more than 30 exercises of varying scales, to test plans in particular offices or specific elements of disease control systems. Some have involved operational partners and the media; others have been more low key with internally focussed objectives. The Department has produced a "lessons learned" report after each exercise including a list of action points which will be incorporated into revised internal instructions and later updates of the main contingency plan. A major exercise, Exercise Hornbeam, was held in June 2004 which involved a Minister, senior officials, many staff from the Department's headquarters and five animal health divisional offices across Britain, as well as other public bodies and stakeholders - altogether more than 500 people. A wide range of industry bodies were invited to attend as observers and their observations sought. Our consultees commented that the value of the Department's exercise could have been increased by including a simulation at farm level, for example to test telecommunications in a remote area.

3.9 The Department's own report on Exercise Hornbeam identified the need for further work. The main points related to:

- changes to roles, responsibilities and organisational structures at senior levels;

- the clarity and presentation of the contingency plan and instructions;

- the need to improve readiness by identifying in advance trigger points for policy decisions during an outbreak;

- improvements to communication systems and procedures; and

- better information collection, sharing and dissemination.

A revised contingency plan will be issued in summer 2005 incorporating the lessons learned from the Exercise.

Vaccination is likely to play a greater role than in 2001, but decisions on its use will depend on circumstances

The contingency plan does not identify a worst case scenario but the Department believes that the plan will cater for most realistic scenarios

PAC main finding: "future [contingency] plans should be based on an analysis of risks associated with Foot and Mouth Disease and should incorporate a range of assumptions about the nature, size and spread of an outbreak, including a worst-case scenario."

3.10 The Treasury minute undertook to further consider a worst case scenario in the light of a revised European Directive on Foot and Mouth Disease. In the event, no guidance is included in the Directive and the Department's contingency plan does not include an explicit worst-case scenario or specify the response to it. The Department considers that its plan should be able to cope with any realistic scenario, particularly as the plan was produced in the light of the 2001 outbreak which is considered by the Department and others to have been an extreme event. The severity of the 2001 outbreak arose from the delay in reporting disease and the silent spread in sheep to 57 widespread premises at a time of the year when there were a large number of sheep movements through markets. However, the British Veterinary Association points out that the virus involved in 2001 did not appear to spread easily to pigs or by airborne means – but may do so in a future outbreak. The Department is now commissioning and contributing to ongoing work with a number of teams to model a wide range of scenarios against which its contingency plans and resourcing arrangements can be checked and developed.

3.11 The Department considers that its plans should be able to cope with any realistic scenario. The variability of the virus, and its likely behaviour in different parts of the country with distinct land holding patterns and densities of livestock, means that the most appropriate disease control strategy, in addition to the culling of susceptible animals on infected premises and dangerous contacts, can only be decided at the time of an outbreak. However, a "Decision Tree", which forms part of the contingency plan, sets out those factors that would influence a decision on which additional disease control strategy to adopt, and this will be augmented as appropriate by the results of the current modelling work.

PAC main finding: "the Department's plans on vaccination should be clear and set out the circumstances and factors that would determine when vaccination would be adopted. The plans should be made known and explained to all relevant parties, including farmers, vets, and representatives of the food industry."

3.12 The culling in 2001 of large numbers of apparently uninfected animals and, in the Netherlands, animals which appeared to have been successfully vaccinated, was controversial. The European Union revised its policy on the control of an outbreak of Foot and Mouth Disease in December 2003 to give greater emphasis to the vaccination of livestock and to allow the animals to live out their normal economic lives. Member states are still required to cull all infected and dangerous contact animals whether or not vaccination is also being used.

3.13 The criteria for deciding whether vaccination will be used in the UK (for example, the size of the outbreak) are set out in the contingency plan and are summarised in the "Decision Tree" **(Figure 8)**. Neither the European Directive, nor most of other countries' contingency plans we examined, contain specific circumstances which would trigger vaccination, and most plans include less detail on how the optimum control strategy is to be decided on. In June 2004, the Department published further details of its vaccination strategy including a number of scenarios where vaccination was likely to be more effective than the basic disease control strategy of culling infected and dangerous contacts. These scenarios include, for example, where a heavily infected pig farm had potentially exposed a large livestock-dense area to airborne spread.

In future, the Department will be able to start vaccination within five days of an initial outbreak

3.14 At the height of the 2001 outbreak, some six weeks after the first case, the Department received permission from the European Commission to vaccinate up to 180,000 cattle in two of the worst affected areas. However, the Department decided against the use of vaccination - mainly due to resistance from farmers who feared that vaccination would be economically damaging.

3.15 In future, preparation of vaccine from stocks of frozen antigen, a process which normally takes three to four days, will begin as soon as the strain of virus causing the outbreak is confirmed. By day five the Department's vaccination contractor can mobilise 50 teams, each of three trained staff, with another 100 teams available immediately thereafter. These teams will allow the Department to carry out a limited vaccination strategy: for example by vaccinating all farms in the 10-kilometre surveillance zone around infected premises to create a firebreak ("ring vaccination"). However, a number of practical problems involved with vaccination remain unresolved.

■ The National Farmers Union fully supports vaccination when recommended on veterinary and epidemiological grounds, but is concerned that restrictions on the sale of products from vaccinated animals may have a significant impact on livestock prices during the epidemic, for which compensation would not be paid. Some farmers might therefore oppose vaccination and prefer their livestock to be culled. The Department is aware of stakeholders concerns over the impact of emergency vaccination on the acceptability of products. The Food Standards Agency has advised that the products of vaccinated animals have no health implications for humans. Nonetheless, food retailers have confirmed that they would not be seeking to differentiate between meat and milk from vaccinated and unvaccinated animals in a future outbreak.

■ The early resumption of exports of animal products (worth some £1.3 billion in 2000) depends on the use of internationally recognised laboratory tests able to differentiate animals that have been vaccinated from those that have been exposed to the virus. Although a number of such tests are available commercially, none have as yet been fully validated and might not therefore be accepted by other countries.

8 The Decision Tree for starting vaccination of animals in the event of an outbreak of Foot and Mouth Disease

Factors influencing the decision of when to vaccinate animals have been set out by the Department in a Decision Tree included in the Foot and Mouth Disease contingency plan.

```
┌─────────────────┐          ┌─────────────────┐          ┌─────────────────┐
│ Can disease be  │          │ Is vaccination  │          │ Are there       │
│ eradicated using│──── No ──▶│ possible?       │──── No ──▶│ additional      │──── No ────────────┐
│ stamping out    │          │     2           │          │ culling         │                    │
│ only?  1        │          └─────────────────┘          │ strategies?  4  │                    │
└─────────────────┘                  │                    └─────────────────┘                    │
                                     │ Yes                         │ Yes                          │
                                     ▼                             ▼                              │
                            ┌─────────────────┐          ┌─────────────────┐                     │
                            │ Is vaccinate to │          │ Are resources   │                     │
                            │ live preferred  │          │ and disposal    │                     │
                            │ exit strategy?  │          │ capacity        │                     │
                            │     3           │── No ─┐  │ available for   │── No ─┐             │
                            └─────────────────┘       │  │ additional cull │       │             │
                                     │ Yes            │  │ strategies?  5  │       │             │
                                     │                │  └─────────────────┘       │             │
                                     │                │          │ Yes             │             │
```

Stamping out of Infected Premises and epidemiologically linked holdings only	Stamping out and vaccination to live	Stamping out and vaccination to slaughter	Stamping out and additional cull strategies	Endemic Foot and Mouth Disease

OIE[1] Country Freedom				No OIE[1] Country Freedom Status until restrictions lifted

Source: Department for Environment Food and Rural Affairs' Foot and Mouth Disease Contingency Plan, Annex D, December 2003

NOTE

1 The Office International des Epizooties (OIE) determines the disease status of countries for the purpose of international trade in animal products.

3.16 In addition, no single vaccine is yet effective against all strains of the virus and the cost of maintaining a bank of vaccines against all known virus strains sufficient for all livestock would be prohibitive. The Department believes that UK vaccine supplies now compare well with European and other developed countries, and is kept under constant review by the Institute of Animal Health, Pirbright, which is also the world reference laboratory for Foot and Mouth Disease. The UK Foot and Mouth Disease vaccine bank holds at least 500,000 doses of each of the 9 main vaccine types and some 20 million doses overall. In addition, there are around 30 million doses covering a wider range of virus strains in the European vaccine bank, which could be made available to the UK in a future outbreak. Some further supplies may also be available from manufacturers, but cannot be guaranteed. A more widespread outbreak than in 2001 may require a substantial proportion of the United Kingdom's 10 million cattle to be vaccinated twice. The UK also has over 40 million sheep and pigs which are susceptible to the disease. However, the Department believes that widespread vaccination of these animals is unlikely to be needed if good biosecurity is practised by farmers. The availability of a suitable vaccine cannot be guaranteed in every case: in the unlikely event that the outbreak involved a new strain of the disease for which no existing antigen was effective, it could take up to eight months or more to produce vaccine.

Culling of animals on infected premises and dangerous contacts will be the main response to a future outbreak, but other disease control measures might also be used

PAC conclusion (ix): "the Department should examine how the contiguous cull was implemented in 2001 and assess its impact and effectiveness, to inform decisions as to whether, and how, a contiguous cull should be used in the event of any future outbreak."

3.17 The 2003 European Union Directive[16] on the control of Foot and Mouth Disease requires the culling of susceptible animals on infected premises and any animals known to have been exposed to the virus by contact with animals, humans or vehicles from an infected place, and allows additional measures to be adopted if necessary.

In future, there will not be an automatic cull of animals on neighbouring (contiguous) premises - unless a potential route of infection is identified by veterinarians. In response to criticisms of the cull policy in 2001 the Department has produced improved guidance on the evaluation of dangerous contacts, including animals on neighbouring farms. The guidance requires the veterinary surgeon attending at the scene to make a judgement on a complex range of criteria. However, if initial efforts to control the epidemic are unsuccessful, and vaccination is not feasible, a more extensive cull of animals on neighbouring farms, as in 2001, remains a possibility because animals on contiguous premises are at greater risk of infection by virtue of their proximity to infected animals.

3.18 The contiguous cull strategy, whereby animals on neighbouring properties were culled premptively during the height of the 2001 epidemic, is still highly controversial. A study in December 2002 by leading academics who advised the Department during the outbreak[17] concluded that, given the widespread and fragmented distribution of disease in 2001, ring vaccination of neighbouring farms would have been a less effective strategy because of the ability of the disease to leap outside the vaccinated area. The study also found that for a wider vaccination policy to be effective it must be started as soon as possible, with cooperation from farmers, and be combined with effective culling of both infected premises and dangerous contacts. It should be noted that this is only one conclusion from a research group that advocated the contiguous cull in 2001.

16   Council Directive 2003/85/EC of 29 September 2003 on Community measures for the control of foot-and-mouth disease.
17   Keeling, M. J., M. E. J. Woolhouse, R. M. May, G. Davies, and B. T. Grenfell, 2003: Modelling vaccination strategies against foot-and-mouth disease. Nature, 421, 136-142.

3.19 The Department made available all its data on the 2001 outbreak to independent academic researchers during 2003. A number of independent studies are underway and one team has published results during 2004 suggesting that the contiguous cull did not have a statistically significant impact on the progress of the 2001 epidemic, but confirming that rapid culling of infected premises was essential.[18] Other academic studies have been critical of the computer models used by various research teams to reach their conclusions. The Department believes that the results of existing epidemiological modelling must be treated with caution and is seeking to improve its existing disease models to allow more accurate testing of alternative disease control strategies. In January 2004, the Department commissioned a major study on the cost-benefit analysis of Foot and Mouth Disease control strategies - the initial results are due for publication in early 2005. The Department's Science Directorate produces an annual report evaluating relevant academic research on Foot and Mouth disease which will be updated in July 2005.

Mass burial pits and on-farm pyres will be used only as a last resort in a future epidemic

PAC main finding: "the Department ...should have not disposed of carcasses on mass funeral pyres."

3.20 In March 2001, burial of culled cattle born before August 1996 was stopped, to avoid the risk that the BSE agent could result in long term contamination of groundwater. Considerable use was made of mass funeral pyres. Although the risk from BSE in a future epidemic is likely to be negligible, the Department considers that on-farm burial or open pyres remain undesirable environmental options and will be allowed only in remote areas or, exceptionally, where no other alternative is available. The Department's contingency plan for Foot and Mouth Disease assumes that disposal of carcasses in a small epidemic should preferably be through incineration or by rendering. However, there is limited surplus capacity in these industries and larger outbreaks will require the use of commercial landfill sites. On-farm pyres, or burial, will be used routinely only in remote areas (for example the highlands of Scotland). The Department is working with the Environmental Services Association to assess landfill capacity across the country.

The Department now has contingency plans for three other major diseases, and internal instructions on notifiable diseases have been revised

PAC conclusion (iv): "Foot and Mouth Disease is only one of a range of serious animal health diseases and the Department will need to look at all its contingency plans afresh in the light of what happened in 2001."

3.21 The Department published in October 2003 a contingency plan for classical swine fever, the most serious disease affecting the European pig industry. In April 2004 the Department laid before Parliament a contingency plan covering two major diseases of fowl (Avian Influenza and Newcastle Disease). These plans are based on the existing Foot and Mouth Disease plan, amended to deal with the particular characteristics of the various diseases. With the exception of Australia, few countries that we examined during the study had published detailed contingency plans for a wide range of animal diseases. In the UK, there are also detailed internal instructions maintained by the State Veterinary Service on each major notifiable disease. The Foot and Mouth Disease instructions are the first to be fully revised and they were placed on the Department's website in 2003.

The Department believes that plans are now in place to engage sufficient resources to control an outbreak of Foot and Mouth Disease

3.22 Prior to the 2001 epidemic, the Department considered that it could control an outbreak affecting 10 farms with the resources it had immediately available within the State Veterinary Service. In the event, where at least 57 farms are believed to have been infected before suspicion of disease was first reported to the Department, the further rapid growth of cases swamped the resources available. The Department has taken steps to ensure plans are in place to deliver sufficient manpower resources, and improved computer support to respond effectively to a future outbreak. The Department's response to specific recommendations made by the Committee on resources is discussed in the following paragraphs.

---

18   Relationship of speed of slaughter on infected premises and intensity of culling of other premises to the rate of spread of the foot-and-mouth disease epidemic in Great Britain, 2001 N Honhold; N.M. Taylor; L.M. Mansley; A.D. Paterson, Veterinary Record, 4 September 2004.

The availability of trained veterinary experts is essential to controlling a major animal disease outbreak

PAC conclusion (v): "the Department needs to decide what measures are needed to increase veterinary resources quickly at the start of any crisis. It should also clarify the basis on which vets recruited from outside would be paid and the terms and conditions on which they would be employed."

3.23 During the outbreak of Classical Swine Fever in 2000 which infected only 16 farms, 80 per cent of the State Veterinary Service's 200 veterinary staff and 25 per cent of its administrative staff were diverted to disease control tasks. During the much larger 2001 Foot and Mouth Disease epidemic, 2,575 veterinarians were recruited from a wide range of sources, including from overseas, in order to deal with the outbreak, but acute shortages remained and other key work such as testing for Bovine Tuberculosis had to be set aside. The Department considers that the need for overseas vets during the 2001 epidemic demonstrated that the existing arrangements were not the most efficient way of using potentially available domestic veterinary manpower. Only a quarter of the 7,000 local veterinary inspectors, private vets who carry out a range of functions valued at £50 million a year on behalf of the Department, carried out any Foot and Mouth Disease related work. The British Veterinary Association considers that this was due to the unrealistic remuneration offered, which is related to the State Veterinary Service salary scale rather than typical fee rates for private practice. However, the Department believes that the majority of local veterinary inspectors specialise in domestic pets, and estimates that some 70 per cent of local veterinary inspectors with farm experience volunteered for Foot and Mouth Disease duties.

3.24 The Department has consulted on plans to create a pool of private practitioners who would be contractually required to undergo training and to give assistance during a future epidemic as contingency veterinary service officers, and to improve recruitment of temporary staff from private practice and retired vets in an emergency. In addition, in May 2004 the Department formalised an agreement with the state veterinary authorities of Ireland, USA, Canada, Australia and New Zealand to provide for the exchange of veterinarians and other experts, such as laboratory diagnosticians and animal health technicians, to tackle notifiable disease outbreaks in any of the six countries.

PAC main finding: "…if the Department commissions a report of vital importance affecting animal health they should implement its recommendations and not procrastinate."

3.25 Many of the problems encountered by the State Veterinary Service in 2001 had been anticipated by an internal study in 1999, the Drummond Report. The Committee of Public Accounts expressed concern that the Department had been slow in implementing the study's recommendations. The Department now prepares a detailed action plan in response to all major studies, including the report on Foot and Mouth Disease from the Committee, and internal audit work. These action plans are subject to regular review and progress reports. For Foot and Mouth Disease, the Department prepared a 'Route Map', which summarises the actions planned to implement the recommendations of all major inquiries relating to the 2001 outbreak. The Route Map is available on the Department's Internet site.

Regional Operations Directors will take up post immediately on confirmation of an outbreak

PAC main finding: "the Department … should have brought senior administrators in earlier to take charge of local disease control."

3.26 In 2001, a need was identified for senior administrative staff to take charge of the disease control operation during an outbreak, so allowing vets to concentrate on matters requiring their expertise. Six members of the Senior Civil Service have been appointed, initially for three years, as contingency Regional Operations Directors, and will take up designated posts immediately on confirmation of an outbreak. In addition, eight Departmental staff have been appointed for three years as contingency Divisional Operations Managers in England and a further seven as contingency finance managers. The Department has established a volunteer's register to identify additional staff likely to be available in an emergency.

The Department and the Ministry of Defence have decided not to prepare firm plans for engaging military personnel in an outbreak

PAC main finding: "working closely with the Ministry of Defence, the Department should define the military's role and identify the tasks it would carry out in any future outbreak. There should be clear trigger points as to when military support is requested and brought into effect."

3.27 The contingency plan provides no details of specific events or circumstances that might trigger military involvement. The Treasury Minute argued that the Ministry of Defence cannot guarantee the availability of troops to assist in any civil emergency because military operations must take priority. The Department has therefore planned to combat an initial outbreak using its internal resources and those of contractors, without recourse to military personnel. The current Foot and Mouth Disease contingency plan requires the military authorities to be notified as soon as an outbreak is confirmed, and the Department has requested that Military Liaison Officers be appointed to National and Local Disease Control Centres immediately they are set up. The Department believes that this arrangement is consistent with the national arrangements for civil contingencies which have been the subject of a recent review by the Cabinet Office[19], that it is now much better prepared for an outbreak than in 1967 or 2001, the need for large scale early military involvement is reduced, and that the contingency plan retains a degree of flexibility to adapt to the particular circumstances in a future outbreak. The Department also believes that the skills which the military brought to the 2001 operation, including the emphasis on leadership and communications, are being maintained within the Department and through regular realistic exercises and by inclusion in the contingency plan. Other areas where military expertise played a major part, such as carcass disposal logistics will be managed through contracts with commercial firms.

The Department is improving its computer systems to allow it to fight epidemics more effectively

PAC conclusion (vi): "the Department needs to develop a reliable computer system to enable it to track the progress of any future outbreak of disease and take swift and effective measures. The system needs to be fully maintained … when there are no disease outbreaks."

3.28 The Department's communications and information systems were severely stretched throughout the 2001 epidemic. Development of an improved web-based database, the Exotic Disease Control System (ExDCS), has been undertaken. This is intended to improve the recording of progress on the key activities associated with control of notifiable diseases of animals, provide management information to staff at all levels and provide links to financial control systems and with the Veterinary Laboratories and the World Reference Laboratory for Foot and Mouth Disease. A prototype system was due to be delivered for assessment by users in June 2004, but plans to outsource the Department's Information Technology resulted in recruitment problems which disrupted development. The State Veterinary Service is now reviewing the ExDCS with the Department's information technology providers to ensure that ExDCS is fully integrated in the State Veterinary Service Agency's information technology programme. The current Disease Control System which was developed in 2001 is being upgraded to ensure ongoing support in the interim and staff training on this will continue.

The quality of senior management in the Department is being assessed independently

PAC main finding: "longstanding attitudes are in need of reform, and the Department's new development programme for senior managers will need to be radical if the necessary change of outlook is to be achieved."

3.29 In creating the Department for Environment Food and Rural Affairs in 2001, the Prime Minister said that it should operate as "a single, distinct and integrated whole, with a markedly new culture". The Department's change programme (*Developing Defra*) is intended to produce major changes in its culture and communications. The programme includes over 100 separate initiatives, including the Senior Managers' Leadership Development Programme which consists of a number of stages including 360-degree feedback, Development Centres and individual coaching. A total of 750 senior officers will have undergone training and assessment by July 2005. A number of the groups we consulted during our study consider that a major, and positive, change in the Department has been evident since 2001.

---

19   Dealing with Disaster (revised 3rd edition) Cabinet Office Civil Contingencies Secretariat ISBN 1-874447-42-X.

PART FOUR
The Department has improved controls over the costs of future epidemics

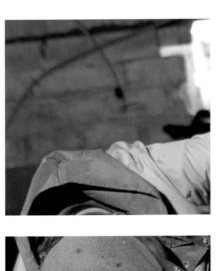
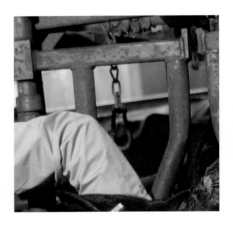
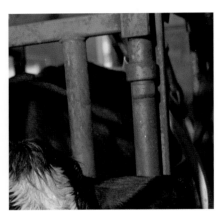
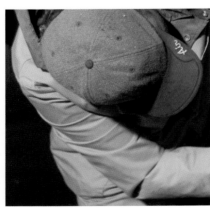
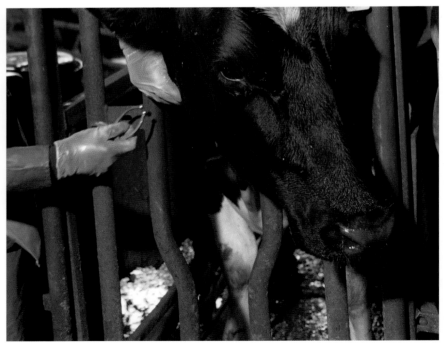

4.1 This part of our report examines the progress the Department has made in responding to criticisms from the Committee of Public Accounts about its control over the costs of an outbreak, especially compensation to farmers and payments to contractors. **Figure 9** summarises our findings on these issues using a traffic light analogy.

9	Traffic light analysis - Controlling the costs of a future outbreak	
Report Ref	**Area**	**NAO evaluation**
4.2-4.8	Compensation for animals is fair	●
4.9	The agriculture industry will share the costs of a future epidemic	●
4.10	A large welfare cull will not be needed	●
4.11-4.13	Procurement of goods and services will be at normal prices	●
4.14-4.17	Cleansing and disinfection costs are controlled	●

KEY

● Committee of Public Account's concerns addressed

● Concerns mostly addressed

● Progress is ongoing to address the Committee's concerns

Source: National Audit Office

A new system of compensation is planned for 2008-09 but in the meantime some issues remain outstanding

PAC main finding: "systems of compensation to farmers for slaughtered animals need to give firmer control over the amounts paid, ... better benchmarks ... and it should not allow potential recipients of compensation to select and appoint the valuers."

4.2 The Department considers that the current legislation limits its scope for amending the compensation system for Foot and Mouth Disease to base valuations on standard values. The compensation regime for Foot and Mouth Disease is prescribed in schedule 3(3)(2) of the Animal Health Act 1981 (as amended). Any changes to this scheme would therefore require primary legislation, which is not likely for some time. The Department is currently proposing to introduce a standard valuation scheme in respect of four cattle diseases on which compensation is currently being paid (Brucellosis, Bovine TB, Enzootic Bovine Leukosis and BSE) as these require only secondary legislation to amend. This consultation constitutes the first stage in introducing longer term proposals for rationalising compensation for all notifiable animal diseases, including Foot and Mouth Disease. In October 2003 the Department consulted on a scheme which would introduce a single system of compensation for all notifiable animal diseases, and avoid the need for animals to be valued individually during an outbreak. For commonly traded types of animal, standard valuations would be published monthly based on actual market information. The information would be updated regularly during an epidemic using indices so that compensation payments would continue to reflect likely market prices. The owners of higher value animals, such as pedigree bulls, would have the option to have them valued at their own expense prior to the outbreak, and the valuation agreed with the Department.

4.3 In the meantime, the Department has improved its existing valuation system for Foot and Mouth Disease. The Department has drawn up a list of 280 approved valuers who will be paid by the hour rather than by a percentage of the valuation as in 2001. The Department has also appointed four "monitor" valuers who will quality assure selected valuations and will be available to advise the Department on any additional instructions and guidance that might be needed to be issued to approved valuers during an outbreak. They would also be available to advise on valuers queries. The Department believes that the valuer system did not work well in 2001 mainly because farmers were allowed to select the valuer. In future any valuer whose methods give significant cause for concern will be removed from the approved list.

4.4 The Department has also revised and updated its guidance to valuers, as promised in the Treasury Minute, and the guidance is significantly better than that provided to valuers during the 2001 epidemic. The Department's published guidance to valuers is now more detailed than those publicly available from most other countries we examined, although the Australian guidance is more detailed again and includes, for example, worked examples and advice on the valuation of high value stud and breeding animals by reference to insurance valuations.

4.5 The Department believes that these interim changes to its system of valuation balance the need to secure value for money whilst ensuring the independence of the valuer. The Department's new guidance expects professionally qualified valuers to be competent. The guidance places more emphasis on typical market prices, but valuers are not required to cite the actual market data being used as the basis for valuation. Nor does the guidance refer to or provide benchmarks as a guide to valuation. However, the Department is aware that there are still a range of factors which can tend to result in over-valuation, particularly for pedigree and higher value animals where there are few open market transactions on which to base a valuation.

Proposals to adjust future compensation to reflect poor biosecurity measures have proved controversial

PAC conclusion (vii): "the level of compensation for farmers should be linked to the adequacy of biosecurity on their premises, and the Department should consider whether a practical scheme could be devised."

4.6 The Department remains concerned that in 2001 too many farmers failed to take even basic preventative animal health measures. In North Yorkshire and Cumbria alone, more than 1,000 investigations were carried out into suspected biosecurity offences. Most of these investigations exposed some degree of biosecurity problem and there were serious breaches in over 70 cases, where formal or informal cautions were issued or court action taken. As part of the Animal Health Bill, the Department proposed to link up to 25 per cent of compensation for infected animals to the adequacy of farm biosecurity. The provision was withdrawn by the Government in October 2002 due to criticism from Members of Parliament that the measure was crude and might prove counterproductive. In June 2003, the Department issued improved guidance to farmers on biosecurity during an animal disease outbreak.

4.7 The Department therefore has no plans to reintroduce proposals for a link between biosecurity and compensation because it considers that it would be difficult to assess biosecurity objectively, and attempts to adjust compensation would lead to frequent legal challenge from farmers. In 2001, the Netherlands reduced compensation payments to a third of its farmers because of poor biosecurity on their farms. The Dutch authorities have now discontinued this policy, but have introduced spot fines ranging from £370 to £3,400 for breaches of biosecurity rules and compensation is also reduced by 50 per cent for infected animals. Animal health authorities in Germany, Australia and the United States continue to have the power to withhold compensation payments in cases where biosecurity rules are breached. The Department's proposals for an animal disease levy are likely to include a variable element linked to levels of biosecurity. In addition, farmers who deliberately and seriously breach biosecurity rules within controlled zones around infected premises will continue to be at risk of prosecution.

4.8 The Department considers that basic disease prevention measures are an essential to livestock health. Although the Department has published biosecurity advice for farmers, it recognises that there is a need to change behaviours and to promote better biosecurity through its work with farmers and livestock associations. In particular, the Department hopes to develop more effective communications strategies for each sector, which will emphasise the economic impact of disease to farm businesses and encourage wider use of farm health plans designed to prevent disease.

Proposals for a scheme to share the cost of a future epidemic between the farming industry and the tax-payer are under development

PAC conclusion (xi): "the Department should report its conclusions to Parliament [on a subsidised insurance scheme or a joint industry-government levy scheme]. "

4.9 The Department established a working group in January 2002 with representatives from the livestock and insurance industries to explore various options to share the costs of future disease outbreaks including compulsory and voluntary insurance as well as a levy scheme. The Treasury Minute promised to hold a consultation exercise on the industry levy in the summer of 2003. However, the exercise has been delayed following concerns of Ministers that the scheme should reflect a clear strategy on the regulation of farming and the cumulative impact of policy changes, including reform of the Common Agricultural Policy. The levy is now part of the broader context of cost-sharing for animal health, under the Animal Health and Welfare Strategy, on which the Department intends to consult as soon as possible. The Department plans to report its conclusions to Parliament following this consultation.

In future, any welfare cull scheme will be limited to a free disposal service

PAC conclusion (xii): "future welfare [disposal] schemes should have clear objectives and eligibility criteria which can be readily checked. Payments to farmers should be set at a level that encourages applications to be submitted only in respect of genuine welfare cases."

4.10 Almost a third of the six million adult animals destroyed in 2001 were culled due to welfare concerns rather than to control the disease. Although welfare compensation rates were set at 80 per cent of the standard valuation[20], concerns were raised during the epidemic that this was generous for the low quality of animal culled under the scheme and that the scheme rewarded farmers who failed to take care of their livestock. The latest contingency plan states that the Department will meet only the costs of the welfare cull and disposal of carcasses, but no compensation will be paid for the value of the animals. Various organisations expressed concern to us about the impact of an extended movement ban on animal welfare and suggested that free disposal alone is unlikely to be attractive to farmers and could lead to severe animal welfare difficulties. The Department believes that other initiatives will help mitigate the adverse welfare effects of movement restrictions and restricted compensation arrangements:

■ A system of licensed movements will allow essential movements to proceed, subject to veterinary advice. Some movements will be allowed in controlled zones around infected premises, mainly to slaughter.

■ The Department will assist the development of a national brokering service to facilitate access to fodder.

---

20   See *The 2001 Outbreak of Foot and Mouth Disease* HC 939, 2001-02, Paragraphs 4.16- 4.20.

The Department is now able to employ approved contractors quickly at pre-agreed rates

PAC main finding: "the Department should negotiate pre-arranged rates and fees for goods and services, which could be brought quickly into use in the event of a future outbreak. Claw-back arrangements should be in place to prevent firms making excessive profits at the Department's expense. A list of approved contractors should be drawn up, and kept up to date, and the capabilities of firms to carry out contracted tasks should be tested in simulation exercises."

4.11 Since 2001, the Department has negotiated agreements (contingency contracts) with a wide range of contractors able to supply the goods and services needed for disease control operations. By April 2004 the Department had concluded agreements with 270 approved contractors to provide the full range of services needed for disease control. The agreements include a standard termination clause and a procedure for resolution in the event of a contractual dispute, including "clawback" arrangements.

4.12 The agreements that we examined reflected current commercial prices. Some, but not all, agreements provide for reduced rates for longer term use, for example the hire rates for vehicles and equipment will reduce after 14 days. Under the Department's contingency plan, specialist procurement staff will be available at disease control centres from the beginning of the outbreak to advise on the agreements and any additional contracting necessary to deal with unforeseen circumstances. In the event of another outbreak, the Department plans to deploy more staff resources to monitor contractors on farm, to minimise the type of contractual disputes that occurred in 2001 (see Part 5).

4.13 Regular desk exercises carried out by the Department's procurement staff have confirmed that contingency suppliers are able, and willing, to deliver the agreed services and equipment at short notice. The Department remains concerned that a major epidemic will inevitably cause some shortages and exert upward pressure on prices and is reviewing the contingency agreements which are not generally binding on either party. More formal contracts involving annual payments have been agreed with over 150 key suppliers which the Department believes would be legally enforceable. In other cases, the availability of benchmark prices and trained procurement staff, and the ability to call on reliable nationwide suppliers to alleviate local shortages, should allow for more effective management of contractors in a future epidemic than was possible at the start of 2001.

The cost of disinfecting farms in 2001 was substantial and the Department needs to consider alternative strategies

PAC conclusions (xiv) and (xv): "improved guidance should be developed on the standards of cleansing and disinfection to be adopted in the event of any future outbreak. The Department should examine the Dutch experience to assess the risks and benefits of their approach [to Cleansing and Disinfection]. The Department should also examine whether in any future outbreak the cost of cleansing and disinfecting could be met by the proposed insurance or levy scheme that is under consideration."

4.14 Foot and Mouth Disease virus can survive for extended periods and must be destroyed by effective cleansing and disinfection or by quarantine of premises for 12 months. Current UK legislation allows the Department to require the farmer to meet the costs of cleansing and disinfection, but this provision was not used during the 2001 outbreak, to ensure a thorough and consistent approach was taken. In 2001 the Department spent around £300 million cleaning and disinfecting more than 10,000 premises – an average of £30,000 a farm. The Department considers that this was cost effective because no cases of re-infection occurred. However, in the Netherlands, the average cost of initial disinfection was between £70 and £550 depending on the size of the farm. Dutch farmers were subsequently required to cleanse their infected premises at their own cost before authorisation to restock was given. No cases of re-emergence occurred in the Netherlands or any of the other countries affected in 2001. In the UK, many farmers were contracted by the Department to undertake the cleansing and disinfection process on their own farms.

4.15 The Department contacted colleagues in the Netherlands both during and after the 2001 epidemic, but no formal report was produced. The European Union however, was critical of the poor financial control exercised over contractors early in the epidemic, the high rates paid and of the large number of hours used in the United Kingdom compared to the Netherlands. The Commission subsequently disallowed 80 per cent of the amount claimed by the Department (see Part 5).

4.16 Other countries including Australia, New Zealand and the United States also use public funds to meet all cleansing and disinfection costs following a Foot and Mouth Disease outbreak – although some of the costs are recoverable through industry levy schemes. In order to share the costs of future livestock disease outbreaks, the Department's levy scheme currently under development (paragraph 4.9 above) is expected to propose to rationalise policy in this area, with the presumption that Government pays for preliminary cleansing and disinfection and farmers pay for secondary cleansing and disinfection. No date has yet been set for implementation of the levy scheme, which will require primary legislation.

4.17 As promised in the Treasury Minute, the Department issued revised internal instructions on cleansing and disinfection in December 2003. These allow for a reduced level of cleansing where infection is not believed to have been widespread on a property and provides some suggested cleansing regimes for such cases. Officials can also require farmers whose property is unusually badly maintained or untidy to make good at their own cost prior to disinfection. However, there are no guidelines available on the maximum cost per farm or the costs which might be appropriate in a variety of circumstances. The Department believes that a maximum cost per farm is likely to become the standard and it believes that its more flexible approach based on fixed price contracts agreed for individual farms will be a more cost-effective strategy.

PART FIVE
The cost of the 2001 epidemic has yet to be finalised

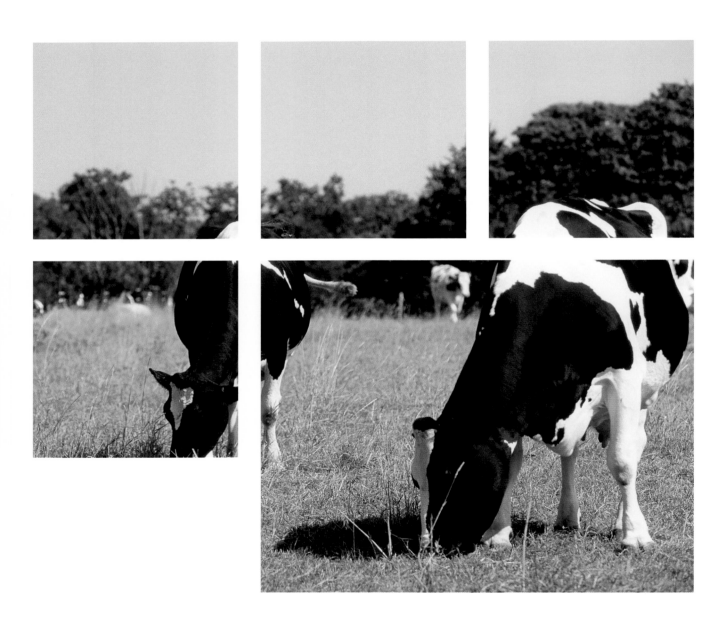

5.1 This Part of our report examines the European Commission contribution towards the costs of the 2001 outbreak, the progress made in contractual disputes with suppliers and the future of the disposal sites used in 2001.

The European Commission concluded that compensation and other costs were higher than necessary in 2001

5.2 The European Union generally contributes towards the costs of disease control in member states. Under these arrangements, the Department claimed a total of £960 million in 2001. The European Commission allowed 36 per cent of the claims. The Department is disappointed with the Commission's findings, which it considers do not fully take into account the unprecedented circumstances of the epidemic. The Department was successful in negotiating a substantial improvement in the Commission's initial offer of £230 million, and has agreed a final settlement of £350 million. More details of these discussions are set out below.

The Commission is to reimburse 39 per cent of the UK claim for compensation paid to farmers

5.3 In December 2002 the Department submitted a claim for £652 million to the European Commission – some 60 per cent of the compensation for animals compulsorily slaughtered during the epidemic (excluding animals culled for welfare reasons). A team from the Commission reviewed the Department's claim and concluded that UK farmers had been compensated for their animals by between two and three times their value in comparison with market prices prior to the outbreak. The Commission concluded that wholesale prices for milk and meat during the outbreak did not support the suggestion that a shortage of animals drove up market prices; indeed prices for most commodities fell during the outbreak. The Commission subsequently agreed to refund £254 million, 39 per cent of the claim.

5.4 The Department considers that the Commission's methodology has exaggerated the extent of over-valuation. The Department investigated a number of cases during the epidemic[21] and commissioned an independent review of farming statistics, market prices and compensation payments. The study identified a complex range of factors which would cause valuations to be higher than expected from market data alone. In particular, the Commission used national average prices for livestock in February 2001 which did not reflect the marked increase in market prices for livestock normally seen during spring, or that market prices in Cumbria are significantly higher than the national average. In addition, as the epidemic continued, a higher proportion of the animals culled were higher value breeding animals or valued with their offspring. These factors were not fully included in the Commission's methodology but the Department concluded that there was insufficient data to be able to estimate the combined effect of all the different factors. A separate review by the Department's internal audit service found that there was a tendency for compensation settlements to be agreed at the top end of its assessment of the range of likely market values. However, legal advice concluded that in the absence of evidence of obvious mistake or deception, there was little prospect of recovery from either the farmer or the valuer.

5.5 The Commission considered that the Department's poor control over the valuation process contributed towards higher than necessary compensation payments. The Commission examined a sample of 100 large compensation awards but found that the rationale for the valuation was largely absent from the files. Its enquiries with farmers and valuers produced explanations which the Commission found to be weak and unconvincing **(Figure 10 overleaf)**. Many of the farmers and valuers contacted by the Commission refused, or were unable, to provide documentary evidence to support claims of pedigree or high productivity.

---

21 See *The 2001 Outbreak of Foot and Mouth Disease* HC 939, 2001-02, Paragraphs 4.5- 4.21.

10 Compensation payments criticised by the European Commission

The European Commission examined a sample of 100 large compensation cases and found that most were poorly documented.

File No. 2 - compensation of £240,715 paid for animals not in fact slaughtered. The Department has recovered this and other overpayments identified by the Commission but has not been able to identify any other cases.

File No. 7 - 317 cattle described as "mostly pedigree bred from top sires" were compensated at an average of £2,035 (compared to an average of £630 paid at English and Welsh markets for dairy cattle in 2000 and the "standard" value of £1,100 offered by the Department). The farmer provided the Commission with certificates for nine pedigree cows, all for animals born prior to 1989, and certificates for bulls unrelated to animals on the claim.

File No. 12 – The Commission queried the valuation of a bull, valued at £30,000, due to its advanced age - a nine year old. The maximum paid at auction for a prime bull in the UK prior to the outbreak was £42,000 – in 1990.

File No 28 - Six rams purchased in October 2000 for an average of £60 were compensated at £535 per head in March 2001.

File No. 59 - 230 milk cows were compensated at £2,940 each due to claimed milk production of 10,000 litres a year. Records produced by the farmer subsequently showed that the farm was 5 per cent above the national average at 6,500 litres per head.

File No. 76 - a farmer paid £14,000 for a yearling bull in January 2001. When slaughtered four months later, the bull was valued at £40,000.

Source: European Commission

NOTE

The Department also investigated a number of cases during the epidemic (See *The 2001 Outbreak of Foot and Mouth Disease* HC 939, 2001-02, paragraphs 4.5 - 4.21).

The Commission is to reimburse 31 per cent of the UK claim for other costs

5.6   The Commission also examined payments for other costs eligible for reimbursement, mainly for the disinfection of farms (see paragraph 4.15 above), but including slaughter feed, rendering, on farm pyres and the destruction of foodstuffs. The Commission agreed to pay £96 million (31 per cent) of the original claim for other costs which totalled £308 million.

It is taking time to resolve disputes with contractors used during 2001

PAC conclusion (xiii): "the Department . . . should seek recovery in those cases where it believes it has been overcharged [by companies invoicing for work carried out]."

5.7   The Department has employed forensic accountants, lawyers, quantity surveyors and other technical experts, at a cost to date of £25.2 million to ensure that invoices from 1,265 contractors totalling £1.3 billion are supported with appropriate evidence. Over 97 per cent of invoiced amounts have been paid but a range of problems has been found on invoices submitted during, and since, the epidemic **(Figure 11)**. In addition to the review of major contractors, the forensic accountants are also reviewing the disputes with the valuers who undertook valuations during the Foot and Mouth Disease outbreak. Twenty-nine valuers accounts are being reviewed with a total value of £3.2 million.

11 Examples of problems found on invoices submitted in 2001

Invoices submitted during the 2001 epidemic did not always meet the Department's requirements.

- contractors unable to supply adequate, in some cases any, supporting documentation to allow an audit of their charges
- inappropriate charges of business overheads, i.e. head office charges
- incorrect application of mark-up rates on subcontracted or supplied materials and plant
- refusal to disclose sub-contractor's rates
- shredding of support documentation
- excessive charges for plant on standby or in use
- sub-standard or alternative materials supplied
- incorrect recording of labour or plant hours
- overcharging for labour/plant time, including charges for travel time
- abuse of accommodation and subsistence provisions
- inappropriate or invalid charges e.g. for personal equipment and tools of the trade

Source: Department for Environment, Food and Rural Affairs

5.8 **Figure 12** shows the progress made in settling contractors' final accounts. Around half the bills by value, invoiced by many smaller contractors, were subject to normal financial controls and have been paid. On the advice of its legal, quantum, technical and accounting experts, the Department initially withheld payment of some £72 million of the £700 million originally billed by 130 major contractors pending agreement of the final sums due. Of the 108 contractors where the Department's investigations were complete at 1 December 2004, a final settlement had been reached in 73 cases. In the settled cases, the Department reduced the original invoiced value of £444 million by £40 million (9 per cent). The Department also believes that it has secured further savings of at least £17 million on the 57 cases on which a final settlement is still to be reached, and some £800,000 through its routine checks on smaller suppliers. In addition, a number of contractors were paid on the basis of estimated costs and the Department is also seeking to reclaim £12 million where it believes contractors were overpaid.

5.9 A total of £40 million worth of invoices arising from the epidemic remain unpaid as at 1 December 2004 due to the time consuming nature of the investigations undertaken and the complexity of the issues. The first two cases to be tested in court were heard during 2003, with the first judgement made in January 2004. In that case, only the first tranche of issues affecting the contractor's account were determined and the majority of these were specific to the contractor rather than having wide applicability. The outcome was a mixed result for the Department. The contractor was successful in claiming some £2.3 million of the disputed invoices, and a further £2 million remained in dispute and a case was scheduled for trial later in the year. The Department obtained permission from the Court to appeal some £580,000 of the initial award but settled the entire dispute by negotiation.

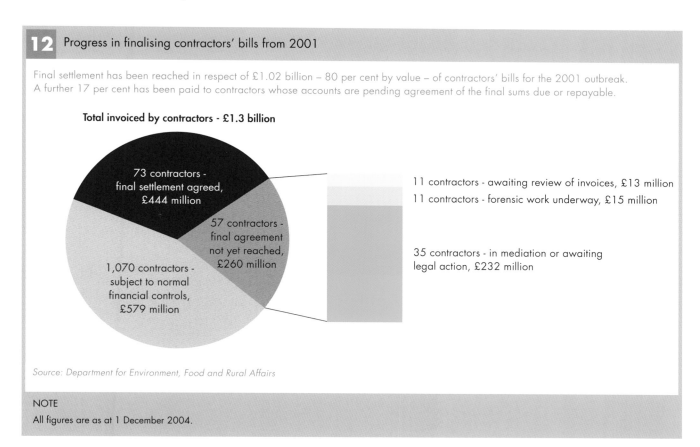

12 Progress in finalising contractors' bills from 2001

Final settlement has been reached in respect of £1.02 billion – 80 per cent by value – of contractors' bills for the 2001 outbreak. A further 17 per cent has been paid to contractors whose accounts are pending agreement of the final sums due or repayable.

Total invoiced by contractors - £1.3 billion

73 contractors - final settlement agreed, £444 million

57 contractors - final agreement not yet reached, £260 million

1,070 contractors - subject to normal financial controls, £579 million

11 contractors - awaiting review of invoices, £13 million
11 contractors - forensic work underway, £15 million

35 contractors - in mediation or awaiting legal action, £232 million

Source: Department for Environment, Food and Rural Affairs

NOTE

All figures are as at 1 December 2004.

5.10 However, the Department considers that the judgement established a number of important issues of principle, which have wider applicability. These include:

■ the Department is not precluded from re-opening paid invoices if errors are discovered subsequently;

■ in the absence of express agreement, a labourer's time and associated operating equipment were not generally chargeable during meal breaks; and

■ weekly summary sheets or timesheets are not conclusive evidence of work done, even when signed by the Department's officers, and can be challenged.

The Department believes that it will be able to use the results of the initial court cases to negotiate settlements in other outstanding cases and is preparing a strategy that balances estimated costs against likely savings in the remaining cases.

Monitoring of mass burial pits will continue for at least 10 years

PAC conclusion (x): The Department needs to formulate plans for the future of each [mass burial] site, and consult local authorities and residents on its proposals. Continued close monitoring and inspection of the sites in particular is essential.

5.11 The Department has undertaken reviews of all seven mass burial sites in Great Britain. It has decided to retain responsibility for management and monitoring the five sites where carcasses are still buried, until there is no significant risk to the environment or public health. This is likely to be at least 10-15 years, but may be significantly longer. Independent contractors carry out regular testing of the sites, and these results are subject to review by the Environment Agency - no significant results have been detected to date.

5.12 Undertakings were given to local residents in 2001 to discuss the future use of the seven mass burial sites that had been constructed. At Tow Law a lease for 70 acres around the main burial site has been agreed with a local Wildlife Trust, at Widdrington the site has been planted with trees and at Watchtree a Nature Reserve has been developed. The Eppynt ranges in Wales have been returned to the Ministry of Defence, and Ash Moor, where no carcasses were buried, will be retained until at least 2009 to ensure that restoration works are effectively managed. A restoration scheme for the Throckmorton site, now known as Ridgeway Grounds has been agreed with the local authority and final capping works have been completed to seal the site. The Birkshaw Forest site in Scotland has also been restored and although the Department retains liability for the disposal activities, the site has now been returned to the landowner.

5.13 Since 2001 some £37 million has been spent by the Department in moving some 150,000 tonnes of ash from 200 farm burial sites where risk assessments have indicated a potential risk to surface water or groundwater. The Environment Agency also monitors the 29 commercial landfill sites used during the 2001 outbreak. Many of these experienced operating problems in 2001-02, including the neighbouring landfills at Distington and Lilley Hall which recorded 63 serious or significant incidents, mainly involving odour.[22] Further public complaints received about these sites since 2001 are not thought by the Agency to be related to carcass disposal. Long term problems are not expected at these sites, but if they did occur they would be a cost to the operator rather than the Department.

22   *Protecting the Public from Waste*, HC156 2002-03, Figure 13.

APPENDIX 1
Study methodology

1   In 2002, the Committee of Public Accounts made a wide range of recommendations for improving the Department's management of future epidemics. We examined:

■   Has the UK introduced cost-effective preventative methods to minimise the chances of a future outbreak of Foot and Mouth Disease?

■   Is Defra well prepared to control a future animal disease epidemic should one occur?

■   Has Defra minimised the costs from the 2001 outbreak (and of future epidemics)?

2   We consulted widely with groups affected by the 2001 epidemic. 34 submissions were received from various stakeholders (Appendix 3 and **Figure 13 opposite**). We also interviewed representatives of: Local Authorities Coordinators of Regulatory Services, British Veterinary Associations, the National Farmers Union, the State Veterinary Service, Veterinary Laboratories Agency, the Cabinet Office Civil Contingencies Secretariat, and the Ministry of Defence.

3   We researched contingency plans drawn up by other State Veterinary Services in USA, New Zealand, Australia, Netherlands, France, Republic of Ireland and compared the UK contingency plan with guidance from the FAO and European Commission Directive on Eradication of Foot and Mouth Disease (Appendix 6).

13	Organisations and individuals who contributed to our consultation exercise

ADAS Consulting Ltd

British Meat Federation

British Meat Manufacturers' Association

British Veterinary Association

Central Association of Agricultural Valuers

Compassion in World Farming

Countryside Council for Wales

Cumbria County Council

Cumbria Crisis Alliance

Devon County Council

Environmental Services Association

Farm Business Advice Service Farmers Union of Wales

Gloucester County Council, Fire & Rescue Service

Institution of Auctioneers and Appraisers in Scotland

LACORS - Local Authorities Coordinators of Regulatory Services

Lancashire County Council

Livestock Auctioneers' Association

Master of Fox Hounds Association

Meat & Livestock Commission

Mr R Miller

National Association of British Market Authorities

National Beef Association

National Farmers' Union

National Milk Records plc

Northumberland County Council

Powys County Council

Ramblers' Association

Royal Association of British Dairy Farmers

Royal College of Veterinary Surgeons

UK Renderers Association

Veterinary Laboratory Agency

VisitBritain

Wales Tourist Board

Mr Adrian Wingfield

4   We carried out a review of scientific academic literature on Foot and Mouth Disease published since 2001 in a range of scientific periodicals including *Nature, Preventative Veterinary Medicine, The Veterinary Record, Research in Veterinary Science, Clinical Microbiology Newsletter, Journal of Rural Studies, Virus Research, Comparative Immunology, Microbiology and Infectious Diseases*, and *Veterinary Journal*. We also liaised with the Royal Society who carried out their own review of the progress made since their report *Infectious Diseases in Livestock* published in July 2002.

5   We also discussed our pre-interim findings with an panel of experts drawn from a range of organisations **(Figure 14)**.

14   NAO Technical advisers

Names	Organisation	Expertise
Tom Hind and Kevin Pearce	National Farmers Union	Chief Dairy advisers, representatives of a major group of rural stakeholders
Keith Sumption	Food and Agricultural Organisation of the United Nations (FAO)	Formerly Lecturer in International Animal Health, University of Edinburgh
David MacKay	Insititute of Animal Health Pirbright	Head of Laboratory and independent scientific expert
Mark Rweymamu	AVIS	Former Head of the FAO Infectious Diseases Group and the EMPRES Programme
Peter Jinman	British Veterinary Association	Ex-President of main UK veterinarian organisation

APPENDIX 2

Sources, signs and impacts of Foot and Mouth Disease

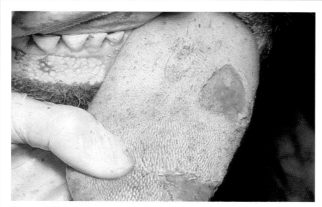

Ruptured blisters on the tongue of an infected steer.

What is Foot and Mouth Disease?

Foot and Mouth Disease affects a wide range of cloven-hoofed animals including three of the most economically important species in the UK: cattle, sheep and pigs. The disease was eradicated from the United Kingdom in the 1960s through a policy of slaughter of all susceptible animals on infected premises and any other animals exposed to the disease.

Where does the disease come from?

Although Foot and Mouth Disease has been eradicated from Western Europe and the developed world, it is still common in much of Africa, the Middle East, Asia and in parts of South America. The disease spreads through movement (sometimes illegal movement) of live animals and through import of meat products into disease free countries. Outbreaks in disease free countries happen from time to time, including major epidemics in the United Kingdom in October 1967 and February 2001, and smaller outbreaks in 1981 and in the Spring of 1967.

What are the signs of Foot and Mouth Disease?

Foot and Mouth Disease is an acute infectious disease. Signs are variable but can include:

Cattle – Fever, dullness, blowing lightly, shivering, sudden reduced milk yield and sore teats in milking stock, tenderness of feet or lameness, quivering of the lips and uneasy movement of the lower jaw with copious frothy saliva around the lips that drips to the ground at intervals. Also, vesicles (blisters) in the mouth, on the tongue, feet, teats and udders.

Source: The Department for Environment, Food and Rural Affairs

Sheep, pigs and goats – Fever, lameness affecting one or more legs, stiff-legged walk, off colour, tendency to lie down and unwillingness to get up, increased mortality in young animals. Mouth blisters are usually small or not visible. (See below).

What are the effects of the disease?

The disease is rarely fatal, except in very young animals. However, abortion, sterility and chronic lameness are commonplace and chronic heart disease may occur. The most serious effects of the disease are seen in dairy cattle as loss of milk yield in subsequent lactations will certainly be experienced and the value of a cow is permanently reduced.

How is the disease spread?

The virus is present in great quantity in fluid from the blisters and in saliva, milk and dung. Animals pick up the virus either by direct contact with an infected animal or by contact with foodstuffs or other things, including people and vehicles, which have been contaminated. Airborne spread of the disease can take place under certain climatic conditions.

Can people contract the disease?

Advice from the Public Health Laboratory Service is that human infection is very rare and causes a mild, short-lived, and self-limiting disease. The Food Standards Agency has advised that vaccination of animals against the disease has no implications for the human food chain.

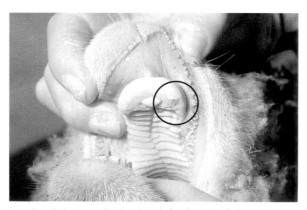

Two day old lesion on the dental pad of a sheep (circled).

APPENDIX 3

Estimated cost of the 2001 epidemic to the Department for Environment, Food and Rural Affairs

Type of cost	Estimated final expenditure (£ million)
Payments to farmers	
Compensation paid to farmers for animals culled and items destroyed	1,158
Payments to farmers for animals slaughtered for welfare reasons	211
Total payments to farmers	**1,369**
Direct costs of measures to deal with the epidemic	
Haulage, disposal and additional building work	375
Cleansing and disinfecting	304
Extra human resource costs	236
Administration of the Livestock Welfare (Disposal) Scheme, including operating costs, disposal charges and slaughter	164
Payments to other government departments, local authorities, agencies and others	89
Miscellaneous, including serology, slaughtermen, valuers, equipment and vaccine	81
Claims against the Department	30
Total direct costs of measures to deal with the epidemic	**1,279**
Other costs	
Cost of the central government departments' staff time	100
Support measures for businesses affected by the outbreak	282
Disposal of ashes from on-farm pyres	30
Total other costs	**412**
TOTAL ALL COSTS	**3,060**
Less: Contribution from the European Commission	(350)
Net Cost	**2,710**

The final net cost of the 2001 epidemic of Foot and Mouth Disease is around £2.7 billion. Some £52 million of invoices are the subject of dispute.

Sources: National Audit Office and the Department for Environment, Food and Rural Affairs

APPENDIX 4

Undertakings given by the Department to the Committee of Public Accounts

The Treasury Minute (Cm 5801 May 2003) sets out the Department's response to the Committee of Public Accounts 5th Report of 2002-03 (*The 2001 Outbreak of Foot and Mouth Disease* - HC 487 of 14 March 2003)

Recommendation (including reference to finding by the Committee of Public Accounts)	Treasury Minute Undertakings	Report reference
On preventing a future outbreak		
... The Department should ensure that the [import] measures adopted in the United Kingdom are at least the equal of those elsewhere in the developed world, including Australia, New Zealand and the United States.	...Public awareness is being raised – through a variety of publicity measures... the first annual report to Parliament due to be published later in May or early June. The final version of the Action Plan will be published in late May... The Government is making £25 million available over the next three years...	6 2.3-2.5
PAC conclusion (iii): ... The Department should aim for a high degree of awareness of animal disease in the farming industry. It should work with other organisations, including those in the voluntary sector, to educate farmers and vets about diseases they might not have encountered, but which nevertheless present a real risk.	... The ... first year of the Veterinary Surveillance Strategy includes the development of a draft "education programme". ... a draft biosecurity action plan... the Department is funding a pilot demonstration farm project, due for evaluation by March 2004... An action plan ...[for farm advice services] by December 2003.	2.2 2.6-2.7
... The Department... should have imposed a national movement ban from the first day; it should have kept the countryside open and not allowed the blanket closure of footpaths for such a long time.	... a GB wide national movement ban of susceptible species will be put in place immediately a case of Foot and Mouth Disease is confirmed and that footpaths will only be closed within the 3km Protection Zone.	6 2.8
PAC conclusion (viii): ... [the Department] should institute effective checks for unmarked animals and penalise those who deal in them.	new legislation this Autumn [2003]. ... A Framework Agreement ... will be rolled out to [local] authorities during the course of this year [2003]...	2.9-2.10
On contingency planning for a possible outbreak of Foot and Mouth Disease		
The... focus on farming interests, important as these are, needs to be complemented by greater recognition of wider rural and national concerns.	... Defra will consult the [Rural Affairs Forum for England] on all important issues affecting the rural economy and rural communities.	8 3.5-3.7

Recommendation (including reference to finding by the Committee of Public Accounts)	Treasury Minute Undertakings	Report reference

On contingency planning for a possible outbreak of Foot and Mouth Disease (continued)

... Contingency plans should not only address farming but also the difficulties likely to be experienced by other industries. ...The Department should bring all interested parties on board and discuss its contingency plans with central and local government, farmers and other major stakeholders. ... The Department also needs to build stronger and more confident partnerships with other relevant bodies in both the public and private sectors, so as to make better use of their expertise and resources (also PAC conclusion (i)).	The Department is actively engaging with stakeholders ... local authorities, police forces, executive agencies, representatives of the farming industry and other rural interest groups. ... Further work is underway to identify and engage with the wider rural stakeholder community to ensure that all relevant industries have had the opportunity to comment on our plans...	7-8 3.5-3.7
Longstanding attitudes are in need of reform, and the Department's new development programme for senior managers will need to be radical if the necessary change of outlook is to be achieved.	... a Leadership Development Programme for all senior managers. ...by July 2004. There will be a review of progress against development plans for all participants, and an evaluation of the impact of the Centre and the subsequent support on individuals' performance and behaviours.	3.29
... Stakeholders ... should participate in the simulation exercises carried out.	A programme of exercises, in local offices, at headquarters and at a national level, is being developed to test the contingency arrangements at all levels. Stakeholders and operational partners will be invited to participate in these exercises when appropriate.	3.8-3.9
PAC conclusion (iv): ... Foot and Mouth Disease is only one of a range of serious animal health diseases and the Department will need to look at all its contingency plans afresh in the light of what happened in 2001.	It is planned that the Foot and Mouth Disease contingency plan will form the framework for contingency plans for other exotic diseases.	3.21

On handling the outbreak

... The Department's plans on vaccination should be clear and set out the circumstances and factors that would determine when vaccination would be adopted. The plans should be made known and explained to all relevant parties, including farmers, vets, and representatives of the food industry.	...A number of issues need to be resolved to make emergency vaccination a fully viable option. Sir Brian Follett suggested this could take 18 months and Defra is working towards resolving these issues, hopefully by the end of this year. ... the Government will make any necessary changes to the Foot and Mouth Disease contingency plan and put in place a communications strategy.	11-13 3.10-3.16
... Future [contingency] plans should be based on an analysis of risks ... and should incorporate a range of assumptions about the ... outbreak, including a worst-case scenario. ... PAC conclusion (ii): Contingency plans must... take account of the risk of an outbreak not being reported promptly...	Further work is underway to develop scenarios on which to assess capacity planning issues in the light of the latest draft of the EU Foot and Mouth Disease Directive which suggests a worst-case scenario.	9, 11 3.10-3.11

Recommendation (including reference to finding by the Committee of Public Accounts)	Treasury Minute Undertakings	Report reference
On handling the outbreak (continued)		
PAC conclusion (ix): ... The Department should examine how the contiguous cull was implemented in 2001 and assess its impact and effectiveness, to inform decisions as to whether, and how, a contiguous cull should be used in the event of any future outbreak.	... On 3 April 2003 the Department announced a call for research proposals ... that investigate the effect of the disease control measures ... Short-term proposals are sought that can be completed in 6-12 months.	14-15 3.17-3.19
It should have brought senior administrators in earlier to take charge of local disease control.	... Members of the Senior Civil Service ... will take up post on confirmation of an outbreak.	3.26
PAC conclusion (v): ... The Department needs to decide what measures are needed to increase veterinary resources quickly at the start of any crisis. It should also clarify the basis on which vets recruited from outside would be paid and the terms and conditions on which they would be employed.	... Consultation on future arrangements, including contractual terms and training, is expected to take place in early Summer 2003.	7 3.22-3.24
... if the Department commissions a report of vital importance affecting animal health they should implement its recommendations and not procrastinate...	For any future report, the Department will have an appropriate timescale for implementation of recommendations that are accepted.	3.25
... Working closely with the Ministry of Defence, the Department should define the military's role and identify the tasks it would carry out in any future outbreak. There should be clear trigger points as to when military support is requested and brought into effect.	... Once informed of a confirmed case the Ministry of Defence (MOD) will offer advice about their possible engagement ... with clear aims and objectives agreed at the point of engagement to reflect the particular circumstances of the outbreak.	10 3.27
PAC conclusion (vi): ... The Department needs to develop a reliable computer system to enable it to track the progress of any future outbreak of disease and take swift and effective measures. The system needs to be fully maintained during periods when there are no disease outbreaks.	...Work is already in hand to develop and introduce a new computer system (the Exotic Disease Control System or ExDCS). ... [existing] systems will be maintained ...The new system should be fully operational in early 2005.	3.28
On controlling the costs of the outbreak		
... Systems of compensation to farmers for slaughtered animals need to give firmer control over the amounts paid. The Department needs better benchmarks for determining the rates paid for animals ... and it should not allow [farmers] to select and appoint the valuers.	A new national list of livestock valuers ... issued with detailed instructions on carrying out valuations. ...consultation this summer on a review of the compensation regime ...The Department is also undertaking a study of the valuations awarded during 2001.	16-17 4.2-4.5

Recommendation (including reference to finding by the Committee of Public Accounts)	Treasury Minute Undertakings	Report reference

On controlling the costs of the outbreak (continued)

PAC conclusion (vii): ... In principle there would appear to be merit in the suggestion that the level of compensation for farmers should be linked to the adequacy of biosecurity on their premises, and the Department should consider whether a practical scheme could be devised.	The Department is ... developing an action plan for working in partnership with stakeholders to promote biosecurity and farm health planning. ... farm assurance schemes [should] encourage a stronger emphasis on biosecurity ... will consider this further.	4.6-4.8
... The Department should negotiate pre-arranged rates and fees for goods and services ... Claw-back arrangements should be in place to prevent firms making excessive profits. A list of approved contractors should be drawn up, and kept up to date, and ... tested in simulation exercises.	The Department has put in place over 150 contingency contracts with firms ... [these] will be reviewed on an annual basis to ensure the contracts reflect market rates and the contractor can still perform at the desired level.	4.11-4.13
PAC conclusion (xiii): The Department... should seek recovery in those cases where it believes it has been overcharged [by companies invoicing for work carried out].	The Department ... is actively seeking to reclaim any monies that have been overpaid through negotiation, mediation, litigation and formal overpayment procedures...	21 5.7-5.10
PAC conclusion (xi): ... The Department should report its conclusions to Parliament [on a subsidised insurance scheme or a joint industry - Government levy scheme].	... A joint consultation exercise ... planned for this summer. Government will report to Parliament on the outcome of this consultation.	19 4.9
PAC conclusion (xii): ... Future welfare [disposal] schemes should have clear objectives and eligibility criteria which can be readily checked. Payments to farmers should be set at a level that encourages only ... genuine ... cases.	...[no] compensation payments to farmers in any future livestock welfare disposal scheme. ... Nevertheless ... lessons will be drawn from the 2001 scheme.	4.10
PAC conclusion (xiv) and (xv): ... Improved guidance should be developed on the standards of cleansing and disinfection to be adopted in the event of any future outbreak ... The Department should examine the Dutch experience ...[and if] the cost ... could be met by the proposed insurance or levy scheme.	Lessons learned during the outbreak are now feeding into a revision of the guidance. ... Government funding of secondary cleansing and disinfection will be subject to review and consultation this summer.	18 4.14-4.17
PAC conclusion (x): ... The Department needs to formulate plans for the future of each [mass burial] site, and consult local authorities and residents on its proposals. Continued close monitoring and inspection of the sites in particular is essential.	... ongoing consultation and discussion with relevant local authorities and community groups to agree restoration proposals and the long-term management. Non-operational sites ... will be disposed of ... At all six sites used for carcass burial ...monitoring will continue.	5.11-5.13
... it should have not disposed of carcasses on mass funeral pyres...	No plans to use mass funeral pyres for the disposal of carcasses.	3.20

APPENDIX 5

Analysis of rural stakeholders' views

Key to those consulted:

A - Auctioneers' Group
AC - Academic
D - Disposal Group
FG - Farmers' Group

FR - Fire and Rescue Service
G - Government Organisation
I - Individual Consultees
LA - Local Authorities

PG - Farm Product Related
RC - Rural Consultant
RS - Rural Support Group
T - Tourism Group

V - Veterinarians
VA - Valuers

View	Further Detail	Expressed by
Britain is better prepared for an outbreak of Foot and Mouth Disease than in 2001	Most of the respondents who expressed a view, complimented the Department … *"There is no doubt that the UK is better prepared to deal with another major outbreak".* However, all recognised that further work was needed in certain areas: *"… this action must not result in apathy on the part of industry, veterinary profession or Government".*	A, LA, FG, FR, PG, T
There has been a high level of consultation with farming and non-farming stakeholders	Most respondents felt that the Department's consultation processes have generally been good and that their views have been taken on board.	LA, D, PG, RS
	"The (consultee's) industry has been involved in a number of consultation exercises and this has been appreciated". However, some respondents felt that their role has not been considered in the contingency plans.	FG, LA, PG, RS
	"The Department is reluctant to consult those who have been most affected by outbreaks". *"… there is no reference to the impact on the UK tourism industry, both in affected areas and in London".*	RG, T, V
The simulation exercises carried out to date have not been adequate	Many respondents commented that insufficient testing of the contingency plan has so far taken place. In many cases, this is because the testing has been of the command structure, and no testing on the ground has taken place. *"Defra should endeavour to involve individual farmers more in their Foot and Mouth Disease practice exercises".*	AC, LA, PG, RS, T, V
A "worst case scenario" has not been considered	All of the respondents who expressed a view were concerned that there was no "worst case analysis" detailed in the contingency plans. *"Contingency plans must, in any case, include a worst case scenario".*	FG, V

View	Further Detail	Expressed by
Britain is still not doing enough to prevent disease entering the country via illegal meat imports	Respondents generally recognised that additional resources had been made available, but most felt that not enough was being done to prevent exotic diseases entering the country. In particular, the lack of public awareness and the low profile of UK controls over importing illegal meat was a major source of concern. Some felt that controls similar to those implemented by Australia and the United States of America could be utilised in Britain. *"The first defence barrier must consist of more than a couple of sniffer dogs at an airport and posters (not always read) warning boat and plane passengers against carrying in meat and meat products".*	AC, FG, G, I, LA, PG, RS, V
Biosecurity on farms and animal welfare has been significantly improved	The view that biosecurity on farms and good animal welfare is important in disease control, and is being addressed effectively by Defra, was held by many respondents. *"Biosecurity on farms now has a much higher profile which has resulted in changes in working practices".*	FR, G, PG, T, VA
	However, a significant minority of respondents felt that the biosecurity measures were insufficient, and did not have the weight of legislation behind them for them to be enforced. Some respondents believe that penalties for poor biosecurity are needed. *"This vital part of the armoury in the fight against disease spread is almost impossible to enforce and relies entirely on farmers' goodwill".*	C, LA, V
The standstill period for livestock movements following the purchase of new animals is adequate	The majority of respondents felt that the six day standstill period was a sensible and balanced policy. *"The adoption of the standstill as a permanent arrangement represents real progress".*	AC, FG, PG, V
	A minority felt that a six day standstill period is not long enough to detect diseases, and that the exceptions to this rule could encourage illegal movements and trading. A minority felt that such a short standstill had no value. *"The reduction of a standstill period (from 20 days during the 2001 outbreak).... raises the question, is there a need for any such standstill period at all?"*	A, LA, PG

View	Further Detail	Expressed by
Guidance on the closure of footpaths during an outbreak is clear and will avoid the closure of the countryside	Most respondents warmly welcomed the revised policy which closes footpaths only around infected premises and limit the damage to tourism that was experienced during the 2001 outbreak. *"We welcome the proposals not to implement blanket footpath closures".*	LA, T
	However, some commented that the guidance could cause confusion amongst members of the public. One expressed concern that the vagueness of the regulations might lead some local authorities to close more footpaths, and keep them closed for longer than is necessary. *"The new protocol may leave a situation where it is difficult to impart a clear message to members of the public about what parts of the countryside are open and what are closed".*	FR, RG, T
The early use of the military is essential to effective disease control	All of the respondents who commented on the role of the armed forces in their response, believed that the military were important for disease control in 2001. Many contrasted the apparent indecision shown by Departmental officials early in the epidemic with the positive attitude shown by the armed forces personnel. *"The military …'should not merely be notified as soon as an outbreak is confirmed…' but should be called into play simultaneously with …the Regional Operations Directors."*	AC, PG
Defra will be able to implement a vaccination policy quickly and effectively	The Government announcement that vaccination would be considered from the start of another epidemic was widely welcomed: *"A properly constructed vaccination programme in which treated animals are not automatically slaughtered but can be retained for future commercial use could also help (to control another outbreak)".* However, some respondents called for more research into vaccine effectiveness and the reliability of tests to distinguish between vaccinated and infected animals. Others expressed concern about the extra time required before the country can be declared Foot and Mouth Disease free.	AC, FG, RC, PG
	A few respondents doubted whether vaccination would be effective in the UK: *"We doubt in any case whether the Department could contain a new outbreak through vaccination unless it were very localised".*	PG, V

View	Further Detail	Expressed by
An improved compensation scheme is urgently needed	The majority of respondents believed that the compensation system had led to unrealistic valuations of animals culled in 2001 and delays in culling infected premises: in particular the introduction of a tariff scheme during the 2001 outbreak. *"…led to a considerable increase in the levels of compensation without having a material affect on the speed of slaughter".* There was widespread support for the new standard tariff compensation scheme proposed by the Department in the Treasury Minute as it could reduce costs and allow the more rapid cull of infected animals target to be met. However, there were caveats that it would need regular assessment, farmers would have to agree the tariff, and clear planning of such a scheme would be necessary: *"An agreement needs to be made with the (farming) industry setting out clearly the appropriate (compensation) rates and how they will be determined".*	C, PG, V
	However, one interviewee expressed concern that a standard tariff would discourage farmers from notifying suspect cases. Another questioned whether the standard groupings proposed by Defra could be agreed with farmers and would not therefore reduce the time between detection and cull.	A, PG, VA

APPENDIX 6

Foot and Mouth Disease contingency planning in other countries

During the study we reviewed the contingency plans for Foot and Mouth Disease prepared by a range of countries and compared these with the plan produced by Defra. The various aspects were derived by the National Audit Office from the European Union Directive on Foot and Mouth Disease (Council Directive 2003/85/EC of 29 September 2003), the model contingency plan produced by the Food and Agricultural Organization of the United Nations (FAO) and from guidance prepared by AVIS, a consortium of groups involved in animal health issues including the FAO, the Institute for Animal Health, Compton and Pirbright, L'Office International des Epizooties (OIE), Paris, and Telis ALEFF Ltd, London. The level of detail included in publicly available documents varies considerably and it was not possible to audit international arrangements. Contingency plans prepared by countries outside the European Union are less likely to comply with our criteria. AVIS consider that the UK plan was one of the better prepared countries in terms of contingency documentation, but that there is still room for improvement in places as shown in the following table.

Key to symbols:-

✓ Contained in plan   ~ Partially included/unclear   ✗ Not included in public plan

Aspect	Great Britain	Northern Ireland	Republic of Ireland	Australia	Canada	New Zealand	USA Minnesota	Comment on UK arrangements
Legal powers	✓	✗	✓	~	✗	~	~	UK contingency plan contains an Annex setting out the general legislation under which statutory powers are available for the control of Foot and Mouth Disease.
Financial provisions	~	✗	✓	~	✗	~	✗	Defra's Director of Finance will liaise with Treasury. Arrangements for obtaining Parliamentary approval are not specifically included. A separate Defra Finance Division contingency plan sets out arrangements for financial controls.
Command structure	✓	✓	✓	✗	✗	~	~	The UK contingency plan clearly sets out decision-making arrangements from the Prime Minister through to local disease control centres.
National Disease Control Centre	✓	✓	✓	✗	~	✓	✓	An HQ will be established at the State Veterinary Service's London office. Initially in a single room, there are plans to extend over two floors for larger outbreaks.

Aspect	Great Britain	Northern Ireland	Republic of Ireland	Australia	Canada	New Zealand	USA Minnesota	Comment on UK arrangements
Local Disease Control Centres	✓	✓	✓	✓	~	✗	✗	Local Disease Control Centres will be established initially in the Animal Health Divisional Offices which are responding to the disease and will expand as necessary. Potential sites for expansion are kept under review.
Permanent expert advisory group	✓	✓	~	~	✗	~	✗	The Foot and Mouth Disease Expert Group has now been established and will meet regularly.
Adequate staff resources identified	✓	✓	✓	~	✗	~	✗	Senior staff have been identified, a Defra volunteers register has been established and agreements are in place for the recruitment of staff from other government departments. Contractors are being identified and agreements reached on price and resource level.
Up to date operations manual	✓	✓	✓	✓	✗	✗	~	Much of the detail in the UK plan is set out in internal Defra instructions. These are fully revised and are available to all on the Defra website.
Detailed plans for vaccination	~	✗	~	~	~	✗	✗	The contingency plan contains a "decision tree" and details of vaccination teams. A more detailed vaccination scheme is to be included in the next revision.
Biennial exercises and staff training	~	~	~	✗	✗	✗	✗	A brief reference is made to the need for regular exercises and some details are given for training of State Veterinary Service staff on exotic disease.
Different scenarios including a worst case scenario	✗	✗	✗	✓	✗	✗	✗	Contingency plans in general do not contain specific policies for outbreaks of different sizes. However, the Australian plan has a specific section on dealing with an extended outbreak (endemic).
Public awareness maintained	~	~	~	~	✗	✗	~	Defra has developed a communications plan which covers emergencies such as outbreaks of Foot and Mouth Disease.
Military assistance	~	~	~	✗	✗	~	✗	The UK contingency plans do not specify the roles to be undertaken by military forces. The Irish plan does specify that the military may be used for the cull of wildlife should this prove necessary.

GLOSSARY

Animal Health and Welfare Strategy
The Department's plans for managing the impact of animal diseases and improving the welfare of animals kept by man, whilst protecting the economic and social well being of people and the environment.

Biosecurity
The precautions taken to minimise the risk that the virus might be spread by those working with livestock and visiting farms, and after infected animals have been slaughtered and disposed of. These include thorough cleansing and disinfection of the person, equipment and vehicles by those working on and visiting farms, minimising inessential contact with susceptible animals and cleansing and disinfecting of premises where animals that had been infected or exposed were present.

Civil Contingencies Secretariat
Cabinet Office branch responsible for coordinating the national response to major incidents and national emergencies where no lead department exists. The Department for Environment, Food and Rural Affairs is the lead department for livestock disease outbreaks.

Contiguous cull
A category of dangerous contact where livestock are believed to have been exposed to infection because of their proximity to a neighbouring infected premises.

Committee of Public Accounts
The senior select committee of the House of Commons. Each year around 40 to 50 reports from the National Audit Office are investigated further by the Committee.

Contingency plan
A plan setting out the Department's proposed response to an outbreak of livestock disease.

Cull
The destruction of livestock believed to be infected, or exposed to infection. Carcasses are subsequently disposed of rather than processed for food (slaughter).

Dangerous contact
Animals likely to have been exposed to infection through contact with other livestock or through movements of vehicles, persons or things believed to be contaminated.

Decision tree
A device included in the Foot and Mouth Disease contingency plan to assist officials in reaching key decisions on strategy in the event of a future outbreak (see Figure 8 on page 23).

Disease Control Centre
A centre set up, normally at the Animal Health Divisional Office, to oversee disease control operations within an Animal Health Division.

Disease Control System
The core database used during the 2001 epidemic containing information on infected premises, restrictions served and actions taken etc. Will be replaced by ExDCS from 2005.

Disinfection (Cleansing &)	Disinfection of infected premises is essential prior to restocking as Foot and Mouth Disease virus remains viable for many months, particularly in wet and cold conditions. Preliminary disinfection is started as soon as infected animals have been culled. Cleansing involves the complete removal of organic matter which can protect the virus and may require the destruction of wooden and older structures/equipment which are impossible to decontaminate. Final disinfection is carried out days to weeks after cleansing, and before re-stocking which can be four weeks after disinfection procedures are completed or 12 months if no action is taken.
Emergency vaccination	Immunisation of susceptible animals commenced after an initial outbreak is confirmed. Normally, vaccination is discontinued shortly after outbreaks cease.
Epidemic	A large number of related disease outbreaks.
Epidemiological model	Mathematical models and computer programmes have been developed for predicting the spread of Foot and Mouth Disease and other epidemics. These can be used to test alternative disease control strategies.
ExDS	Computer database under development which will provide a high level of up to date information on the progress of a future livestock epidemic.
FAO	United Nations Food and Agricultural Organization.
Hefted sheep	A flock of sheep acclimatised to local conditions with innate knowledge of local pasture and shelter.
Infected Area	An area of a minimum of 10 kilometres around an infected premises in which strict movement and biosecurity restrictions are in force.
Infected Premises	A farm, or other location with livestock, where Foot and Mouth Disease has been confirmed on the basis of clinical findings by a veterinary surgeon or positive laboratory tests.
Outbreak	Is used in this report to mean a farm or other agricultural location where one or more animals is infected with Foot and Mouth Disease virus.
Protection Zone	The area within a three kilometre boundary of infected premises.
Rights of way closure	Closure of footpaths, normally restricted to 3km around an infected premises (see also protection zone).
Regional Operations Directors	Senior Civil Servants who, from 19 March 2001, were sent to certain Disease Control Centres to manage non-veterinary activities, such as slaughter and disposal, and organise the administrative input.

Ring vaccination

Immunisation of susceptible animals against a disease in a limited area around a confirmed outbreak, intended to create a firebreak preventing the spread to uninfected areas.

Route Map

The Department's proposals for implementing the recommendations made by inquiries into the 2001 Foot and Mouth Disease epidemic by the Royal Society and Cabinet Office. The map also contains a summary of progress made.

Stamping out

The control of livestock disease by the cull of infected animals and those animals exposed to the disease.

State Veterinary Service (SVS)

The UK agency responsible for dealing with notifiable livestock diseases, carrying out welfare visits to farms and markets and advising farmers on disease prevention and requirements for importing and exporting.

Surveillance Zone

The area lying between three and 10 kilometres of infected premises.

Swine Fever (Classical)

A highly contagious viral disease of pigs generally results in high levels of deaths. The disease was eliminated during the 1960s but large outbreaks occurred in 1986 and 2000 due probably to infected meat imports.

Treasury Minute

Government response to a report by the Committee of Public Accounts.

REPORTS BY THE COMPTROLLER AND AUDITOR GENERAL, SESSION 2004-2005

The Comptroller and Auditor General has to date, in Session 2004-2005, presented to the House of Commons the following reports under Section 9 of the National Audit Act, 1983:

		Publication date
Agriculture		
Foot and Mouth Disease: Applying the Lessons	HC 184	2 February 2005
Cross-Government Reports		
Delivering Public Services to a Diverse Society - Report	HC 19 - I	10 December 2004
- Case Studies	HC 19 - II	10 December 2004
Culture, Media and Sport		
UK Sport: Supporting elite athletes	HC 182 SE/2005/9	27 January 2005
Education		
Skills for Life: Improving adult literacy and numeracy	HC 20	15 December 2004
Law, Order and Central		
Reducing Crime: The Home Office Working with Crime and Disorder Reduction Partnerships	HC 16	1 December 2004
Home Office - Reducing Vehicle Crime	HC 183	28 January 2005
National Health Service		
Patient Choice at the Point of GP Referral	HC 180	19 January 2005
Reforming NHS Dentistry: Ensuring effective management of risks	HC 25	25 November 2004
Public Private Partnership		
English Partnerships: Regeneration of the Millennium Dome and Associated Land	HC 178	12 January 2005
Revenue departments		
Inland Revenue: Inheritance Tax	HC 17	3 December 2004
HM Customs and Excise: Gambling Duties	HC 188	14 January 2005
Transport		
Tackling congestion by making better use of England's motorways and trunk roads	HC 15	26 November 2004

Printed in the UK for the Stationery Office Limited
on behalf of the Controller of her Majesty's Stationery Office
176146   02/05   65536